East to West

Dr Thomas Abraham

Copyright © Dr Thomas Abraham, 2020

A contribution from the proceeds of this book will be donated to The Homeless & Rootless Project, Hull; Kerala Forest Development, India; Our Lady of Lourdes Hospital, Pacha, India.

Dedicated to

My father Thomas who was the light of my life

&

My daughter Teresa who was the hope of my life

Contents

Prologue

I was born in India, shortly after Britain left its richest and prime colonial asset by granting independence. My childhood moulded among the mist and midst of British plantations. After qualifying as a doctor, I worked in India for a few years, left for Africa and settled in the UK. I have rendered over three and half decades of service to the NHS.

In the ever-changing society, I did my best to balance the scales of giving a fair trade of my profession, stood up for my brethren and felt obliged to raise my voice against unjust maneuvers from various sources. The driving force in my life has always been the belief that we all belong to not just same Family but same Species *Homo sapiens* irrespective of race, colour, religion or other differences. The verbatim meaning 'wise man' is pertinent and poignant; we all are wise- gifted with different skills, capabilities and qualities. By working together we can process and progress the fabric of the framework of the community, society and humanity.

I was struck down following the tragedy of the death of my daughter. After falling down, I got up and started walking. While limping, there was an attempt to run me over and finish me off. When struggling to survive under deep grief, within a week of funeral of my daughter, two Asian colleagues, one from my own medical school, incited by personal vendetta and professional jealousy, invented and fabricated allegations relating to family matters of bygone days discrediting my unblemished career and condemning my fitness to practice, to cause professional homicide by depriving me, the sole breadwinner of my livelihood and targeting the end point of total disintegration of my family. Eminent doctors, patients and the Community of Hull stood up to support me. At the General Medical Council hearing, justice prevailed. The wounds and scars within me remain unhealed and raw.

Throughout my professional life, I have been listening to fellow human beings in their role as patients not only with their stories of distress, unpleasant experiences and ailments, but also shared the pleasantries of human nature and values and learnt a lot from them. My policy of shrugging off the trappings of formalities in consultations leading to effective catharsis of vital health matters, has paid rich dividends. Interaction with patients have incited revitalization and rediscovery of my inbuilt perceptions and conceptions about medicine and life in general. I feel it my solemn onus and obligation to tell the world of my experiences- pleasant, pungent and painful, because they reflect and resonate on a daily basis with the fundamental realities of life. Most importantly, the truths have to come out and stay open for the common good of the society.

In 1982, Prince Charles, addressing the British Medical Association, commented " ...the whole imposing edifice of modern medicine, for all its breath-taking success, is like the celebrated Tower of Pisa, slightly off balance." Having worked in the NHS over three and half decades, my sentiments are also of a similar nature.

I am encouraging every reader of this book to put pen to paper and jot down because everyone can contribute something to humanity by sharing their life experiences, however small or large.

'Everyone can be great because everyone can serve'.

Martin Luther King

1

Early Years

'If you carry your childhood with you, you never become old.'

India got independence from Britain in 1947. Many British estate owners stayed on for nearly another decade or so. Peermade in the state of Kerala, Southern India was one of the favourite spots of the British. It was a bewitching hill station pure and pristine with rolling hills, wandering streams and gurgling waterfalls. Due to the nice cool climate being 3000 feet above mean sea level, the town is blessed with green canopy throughout mixed with plantations of coffee, tea and cardamom. I was born there as the middle son. My father was a forest officer who worked away. So, I spent most of my early childhood with my grandparents. My mother lived about 100 miles away and my elder brother stayed with her.

In AD 52 St Thomas, the disciple of Christ, arrived in a boat on the west coast of Kerala. He went to a nearby town called Palayoor. The Hindu priests were praying, standing in the water and throwing water up to please the *Sun God*. Watching the scene, St Thomas commented that the water was coming down since God was not accepting it. After making a deal with them, he threw water up and it stayed in the air. That miracle led to their conversion to Christianity. He founded the first church in India there, followed by six others. St Thomas is the apostle of India; his remains are at St Thomas Mount, a small hillock in Madras.

Our house was two-storeyed, sandwiched between a road at the front and a river at the back. The back garden was a place of tranquillity, peace and fun. There were mango trees and a variety of fruits were grown - bananas, oranges, apricots, grapes and passion fruit. My grandmother used to warn me on a daily basis not to drop my guard because poisonous snakes also used it as their sanctuary.

My grandfather had a shop. Punctuality and smart dress were his prime assets. He would call me on the way to school and comment that if he could see his face mirrored while looking into my shoes he was happy. After finishing school, I used to spend time with him keeping him company in the shop and doing my homework there diligently. On finishing my homework, he used to give me a piece of chocolate as an incentive. Lots of my school friends were British, since many of the plantations were owned by the British and stayed for many years after India got independence from British rule.

I used to go with school friends to the mountains during school holidays and play football and lazily loiter eating guava fruits which were in abundance.

One day, on returning, my grandmother noticed blood on my leg. She started questioning me whether I had been fighting with my friends. When I saw streak of blood on my leg, I was alarmed. Grandma took me to the shower and to my horror, I found a leech had gone into my box office. Frightened, I ran out of the bathroom screaming. My grandfather sorted things out. After that, when I went to mountains, I had to wear long trousers and boots. A few months later, a few of school friends senior to me went mountain hiking on a Sunday. Unfortunately one of them went missing. The news spread like wild fire. Lots of men from the town formed a search party and went to the mountains, searching in various directions. They searched most of the night and finally found a python resting after a heavy meal. They caught the python and cut it open to find that it had swallowed a nine-year-old boy, the missing school friend. Tragedy for all of us in the community. I was never allowed to go to mountains anymore.

Over the Easter holidays, my father, mother and elder brother came over for a few days. Being the most junior, I lost my bed and had to sleep on the floor. On the second night about 2 o'clock, I heard a loud scream and something wet and slimy landed on my neck, which I threw, instinctively, and screamed my head off. My father came running from the next room and put the light on to find that it was a very poisonous snake called 'Anali'. It was about two feet long, greyish body with white markings. If it had bit me, I would not be here writing this now. Many British shops were still operating at that time and I had a penchant for 'made in England' goods.

At the age of eight, I moved to Periyar, a wildlife sanctuary, since my father was posted there. It was in the mountainous Western Ghats of Kerala. This wildlife sanctuary is home to tigers and a significant elephant population, as well as rare lion-tailed macaques, sambar deer, leopards and Indian bison. In the park's north, Periyar Lake was popular for boat rides. Farther north, spice plantations surrounded the town of Kumily.

The accommodation was within the forest with trenches around so that wild animals wouldn't come into the house. I remember the elephants walked past at night. One night, an elephant was looking at me when I was studying with bright lights on. I saw him pausing and watching me. From his demeanour I knew that he was very curious and friendly. I went into kitchen and threw some bananas which he enjoyed. Then, as a routine, he would come around most nights at the same time. I did not disappoint him either. I kept my friendship away from my mother. But she said I was eating lot of bananas for my age and it was not good. Eventually I admitted my friendship. So, she got lots of bananas and she also joined the gifting encounters.

2

Backwaters

*'But these backwaters of existence sometimes breed, in their
sluggish depths, strange acuities of emotion.'*

Edith Wharton

At the age of ten, we moved to Edathua, which is in
Kuttanad, otherwise called the '*Rice bowl of Kerala*'. The
place is part of backwaters with interlinking, tranquil
canals and lagoons, fringed on banks by a retinue of
palm trees. The house was in the village surrounded by
green paddy (rice) fields. We had almost everything
grown at home. There was banana plantation and
nearly one hundred coconut trees. Some trees were
designated to draw palm wine *(toddy)* which would taste
almost like champagne. The specialist who would
climb the coconut trees to pluck the coconuts was
called *mannan*. They were experts in that trade, some
would climb 50 trees in 4 hours. Most of these
technicians have now stopped working and the newer
generations do not want to follow the footsteps of
their forefathers because they don't need to for
financial and social reasons. Man being as innovative as

ever, nowadays, people have trained their forefather's forefather to do the job. Man has trained monkeys to do the job of climbing the coconut trees and pluck the ripe coconuts. Time is the key. Some people ride the scooter with the specialist monkey sitting on the back.

The house was in a village, with an acre and half of land, surrounded by rice fields. We had two dogs - a German Shepherd for outside duties and a Golden Retriever for indoor duties. There were cattle, sheep, ducks and chicken. There were lots of coconut and mango trees. The banana plantation had coffee, pepper, passion fruit and a variety of vegetables. Inevitably, poisonous snakes were in residence as well. Cobra was the most common, with hollow fangs fixed to the top jaw at the front of the mouth. They cannot hold their fangs down on prey so they inject venom through their fangs, They have an excellent sense of smell and night vision. They usually prey on rats but do not mind delicacies like baby chicks. My mum used to warn me not to hang around near the chicken shed because the snakes would sneak in to steal the eggs. Two boys had died of snake bites in the village over those last few years.

On the banks of the River Pamba in Alapuzha lies a marvellous structure that is often compared to the medieval behemoths that adorn Europe's landscape. The Edathua Church is famous for its structural prowess and is a symbol of God's Own Country's architectural heritage. Built in 1810, it was dedicated to St George and draws in large crowds for its annual festival (*Perunnal*) of St George. This joyous event occurs between 27th April and 7th May every year and is celebrated with much pomp and flare. A statue of the saint, decked in gold, leads a procession that ends at the Basilica itself. Prayers are offered as the landscape is peppered with a multitude of cultural fêtes and feasts. The interior of the church closely resembles St Charles Borromeo Church, in Jarratt Street, Hull. Other Christian institutions were the Georgian public school and St Mary's Church, Niranom, 6 miles away, which was founded by St Thomas in AD 54. St Aloysius School, which I joined, was very nice. It was a boys only school. The only consolation was the girls' school was round the corner. So, we used to hang around at the gates watching our fairies go past with glances of mutual (sometimes one-sided) admiration. I enjoyed my time there.

As usual, I used to go to the nearby river to bathe daily. One day, during monsoon season, the river flow was very fast and with high tide. When I got into the river, something bit my leg. There was a sudden accent of anxiety and I felt short of breath. In that panic, I gulped some water and lost my footing, lost control and the fast tide swept me away. I started shouting and waving but the words got stuck. A feeling of imminent death dawned upon me. I had been swept nearly quarter of a mile. Then I saw one of my neighbours, Mary, returning home with a shopping bag walking on the river bank in my direction. When she saw me, she jumped into the river and pulled me to safety. Frightened, I fumbled my way back home in a state of disarray. When I told my mum what happened, she nearly passed out. I was grounded; no more bathing in the river.

It was monsoon season. I was 11. After school, my class mate, friend and neighbour, Mathew, was with me. He was not very well. So we went to the compounder (pharmacist) and got some pink medicine for coughs and cold. He drank it. We got on the bus to get home. We normally got down two furlongs before home because that was the limit of a 40 paisa ticket. When we reached there Mathew was nodding off. There was thunder, lightning and torrential rain. We did not get down there. After two stops, we got down and walked home. We both got drenched.

That weekend, on Sunday morning at about 8.30, I was returning after collecting milk. My dad was sat outside reading a newspaper. He asked me, "Did you dodge the 10 paisa fare on the bus?" I was bewildered. Then I paused a bit. I presumed the conductor had reported it to the bus owner, John, who was a distant relative of mine. He asked me again. The more I tried to explain, the less he was willing to listen. Dad said, "How much money have you got?"

I said, "Three rupees and 20 paisa." He said, "Come on, give all the money to John, apologise to him now." It was a strict order. On the way to Uncle John's house, I thought it was a bit harsh, I could give him double the amount - 20 paisa - anything more is not just. In fifteen minutes, I reached Uncle John's house. He was reading a newspaper lying on an easy chair in the porch. He had an unconcealed expression of astonishment as he fixed his eyes on me which seemed to ask, "Why are you here?"

With an affected assumption of fear and doubt, I tried to explain to him what happened on the bus. He was also not keen for any excuses. I just wanted to run away from the scene after giving him all my money. When I gave him the money, he said, "Is that all you have?" I thought in my mind, 'What a greedy uncle, you are filthy rich, why are you squeezing me out of my pocket money?' I apologised and left immediately. When I reached the gate, he called me back. He said he would drop me at my house in his car. I had no choice and reluctantly got into his car. He was unusually quiet. When the car reached my gate, he stopped and got out. Then he said, "By what you have done, you have brought shame on your dad; I don't expect this to happen again." Then he gave me a hug and an envelope. 'You can keep this,' he said. I thought he was giving me my money back. I didn't open it and went into kitchen and had breakfast. A few minutes later, I opened the envelope. A note was written in red, the tenth commandment - **YOU SHALL NOT COVET** - and 20 Rupees. I couldn't believe all that. Later my dad told me, "If you cheat the market trader, God will cheat you. Morals make the man." I felt ashamed and learnt a lot with this stake of 10 paisa.

My local church library was managed by retired priest Fr Michael. He was very friendly and I used to take books frequently; I used to do a lot of reading. When I was 12 years old, one day, I was summoned by the headmaster. He said,

"Two teachers have complained about you."

I replied, "What is it about, Sir?"

"Have you got *The Complete Works of Shakespeare*?"

"Yes."

"There is only one copy in the school. The English teachers need it."

"Ok, Sir, I will return."

I returned the book to the library. Later at the summer vacation, I borrowed it and read it completely. The librarian might have informed the headmaster; I received a letter of appreciation from the headmaster stating that I had read *The Complete Works of Shakespeare*.

3

College Boy

'Twenty years from now you will be more disappointed by the things you didn't do than by the ones that you did do. So throw off the bowlines. Sail away from safe harbor. Catch the winds in your sails. Explore. Dream. Discover.'

Mark Twain

At the age of 14, I passed my Secondary School Leaving Certificate examination in First Class. Then I joined St Berchman's College at Changanacherry, which was 15 miles away from home. I stayed at St Joseph's Hostel here. The hostel life was very regimental. Study and leisure times were very strict. I used to train as a 100 metres runner and play squash and football.

Daily at 5 AM, I and my friend Raju used to run 3 rounds over the football ground. One day, a third runner joined us and started chasing us - a stray dog. Fortunately, we climbed over a nearby mango tree and stayed there eating and throwing mangoes at the dog to chase it away. The dog kept staring and barking at us and refused to leave. At dawn, a batch of ladies going to church, saw our predicament, started giggling with humour and got the watchman to chase the dog away. There were cases of rabies at that time and we decided not to do any more running.

Fr Joseph, the warden of the hostel was humble, sanctimonious, vassal and well-respected. He was very regimental in all dealings. He was a role model for us all. Later on he became Archbishop. He used to celebrate mass at 5 AM. I and my friend, Jonathan, volunteered to be altar boys. We had to pick up wine and water from the back of the altar during the mass. One day, we decided to taste the wine before bringing it across to the altar. After the mass, I felt guilty of pilferage. On the way back, Jonathan told me that in the wedding of Cana, Jesus turned water to wine for all to enjoy. So, we found a lame excuse to justify our actions. We tried it another day. After the mass, Fr Joseph commented with a grin, "The wine tastes different." Our 'wine tasting' came to a grinding halt.

Warden Fr Joseph went away for a week and we went to the cinema. The warden from the adjacent hostel took a sudden roll-call; both me and my elder brother were missing and charged with a third degree offence of eloping – leaving hostel without permission after 6 PM. I had gone to a cinema in the neighbouring town; so did my brother. We both ended up in front of the principal of the college, were given a good telling off and the matter was resolved with an apology and reassurance that the offence won't be committed in future.

Back near my house, some of the bridges on the roads were not completed. Ferries transported vehicles and people across. Most of the daily errands were conducted by travelling on small canoes. One of the most important events was the boat race in Alleppy, which was 15 miles away from my house. This is the equivalent of the Grand National. India's first Prime Minister Jawaharlal Nehru visited Alleppy in 1952. Locals gave him a robust, rousing and rapturous reception by sailing him in a snake boat accompanied by many other similar boats. On conclusion, he donated a rolling trophy – a replica of a snake boat in silver on a wooden abacus. The tournament was later named after him as the Nehru Trophy.

The boat race was held on the second Saturday of August every year in Punnamada Lake. The boats were 100-120 feet long canoes made of wild jack wood (*Aanjali*) carrying 90-110 rowers. The rhythmic rowing mimics the movement of snake. Hence they are called snake boats. The course of the racing track was 0.9 miles. Alleppy is a coastal town near the Arabian sea, with mainly fishing and coir industry. It has a beautiful lighthouse which is 137 years-old. But it also the site of a blood bath in 1946, in the two neighbouring villages called Punnapra and Vaylar. An uprising against the British rule cost 350 lives – a very poignant and painful pointer of past.

I passed the Pre-degree Examination in First Class and applied for admission to medical school. I duly got selected, as anticipated, since it was on the merit of the grade of the qualifying examination. But I was only 16. The minimum age to join medical college was 17. So I had to wait to join next year. I applied to St John's Medical College, Bangalore. I got selected. But I had to do a one year Pre-Professional Course which meant the same end result at both schools.

Trains were very fast and convenient. The overnight sleeper journey took to Bangalore by 7.30 in the morning. Bangalore (now called Bengaluru) is the capital of India's southern Karnataka state. The centre of India's high-tech industry, the city is also known for its parks and nightlife. By Cubbon Park, Vidhana Soudha is a Neo-Dravidian legislative building. Former royal residences include 19th-century Bangalore Palace, modelled after Windsor Castle in England, and Tipu Sultan's Summer Palace, an 18th-century teak structure. The city is famous for being the Silicon Valley of India, It is a well-known IT hub and some of the world's major IT corporations operate out of the city. My dad talked to me about both medical schools and waiting another year before joining. Bangalore was in a different state (450 miles away) and a lot more expensive. So I decided to wait and join medical school in Kerala next year. Looking back, it was a wise decision; as a teenager in a vibrant city far away from home, I might have lost my direction.

4

Medical School Days

'The (medical) student often resembles the poet - he is born, not made.'

William Osler

Getting admission into Trivandrum medical college was an exhilarating experience, akin to winning a 5000 metre race, producing similar addling effects. My qualifying examination certificates were securely curled in a wrapper in my bag. The sudden importance of a being a budding doctor, instilled an aura of intoxication.

Trivandrum (now called Thiruvananthapuram) is the capital of the southern Indian state of Kerala. The word meaning is 'City of Lord Ananta'. It is distinguished by its British colonial architecture and many art galleries. It's also home to Kuthira Malika Palace, adorned with carved horses and displaying collections related to the Travancore royal family, whose regional capital was here from the 18th–20th centuries. The Victoria Jubilee Town Hall, Napier

Museum and Kowdiar Palace are famous attractions.
The Kerala state animal is the elephant and the state
bird is the Great Hornbill.

I set off by train. On boarding, an awful strangeness
descended onto me. I started speculating the possible
ailments of people around me. An elderly couple was
sat opposite me, sipping coffee with monotonous
regularity. They stuck to serene silence, with sporadic
genteel smiles. The uneven roofs of the houses
appeared as a haze due to the speed of the train, like
being engulfed in cotton wool. Pungent nostalgia set
in; the horizon appeared remote and transforming.

I got a taxi and reached the college well ahead of time.
As I walked in, the congregation of all nationalities (we
had system where 5% were foreign students) depicted
the spirit and image of United Nations. There was a
fierce flood of facts and fiction spreading like field-fire
across the corridors. All the students were ushered into
an oak-panelled hall which was systematically
decorated with prestigious portraits of past masters of
the profession. The warm breeze congealed outside,
made an abrupt influx like an unwelcome intruder
disturbing the stillness and harmony. A grandfather
clock in the hall chimed nine times in unmistakable
terms.

The great man, the principal, breezed into the hall.
Silence and patience filled the hall. The principal (head
of the college) was Dr Thangavelu. He was a reputable,
internationally known doctor. The moment he entered
the podium, we felt like going into a trance. He

appeared a sound, singular and solitary stalwart. He extended a warm welcome and gave a general overview of the college, course and curriculum. He quoted Aristotle – 'Men are called healthy in virtue of an inborn capacity of easy resistance to those unhealthy influences that may ordinarily arise; unhealthy in virtue of the lack of capacity.'

He pointed out that when we pass out, we would be heading to all corners of the globe. So, we needed to be aware of our roots and be good ambassadors of the profession. He cited India's glorious contributions to the world. India gave the world first university at Takshashila in 700 BC, with 10000 students, 300 lecture halls, laboratories and an observatory. Cataract surgery was started by Sushruta in the 6th century BC. Plastic surgery was started in 2000 BC. India clothed the world by cultivating cotton in 5000 BC. Before that, animal skin was the fashion to cover modesty. Ayurveda, a complementary and alternative medicine was started in India in 1000 BC and is practised globally now. In the 7th century, Bhaskaracharya calculated the time taken by earth to orbit the sun. India gave the world zero, the decimal system and quadratic formula.

Wearing the white coat gave an aura of being a talisman. Following that, we had a guided tour of various departments. Like a herd of sheep, we were shepherded by various teachers into different departments in classical harmony, culminating in lunch.

We were given time off after lunch, to start the next morning in full swing.

Dr Thangavelu was a real role model. He was very hardworking and would appear from nowhere and when least expected. So everybody was on their toes all the time. With his radiant smile he would stop and talk to anybody- doctors, students, nurses, cleaners and patients. He will put everybody in their place. One day, while I was walking past, I noticed a patient was smoking sat near the pavement in the shadow of a small tree. After finishing the *bidi* (locally rolled cigar) he threw the stub indiscreetly and spat. Dr T was on his stroll. He gave a firm talking through regarding the dangers of smoking, the safe disposal of waste and the hazards of spitting in public places. One afternoon, I was going fast on my newly acquired bicycle down the hill to a physiology lecture which was at the far end of the campus. I saw one of my lady classmates walking; I slowed down with a view 'to show off my new bike' and rode slowly chatting with her. Dr T was coming across. We both greeted him. "Good afternoon, Sir." With a broad smile he quipped, "It is a nice bike; flirting is fine, but mind the road and the speed." He had a great sense of humour.

His roles were, head of the college, teacher, counsellor, supervisor, enforcer-in-chief, de-facto policeman, guide and philosopher. He was an icon of achievements in various aspects, a self-made stalwart. He was an acute strategist who connected the dots and somebody who could see the forest from the trees. His nickname was

'Thungan'. He insisted on a long, lanky, full sleeved, fully buttoned, white coat for all doctors and students; we named it 'Thungan Coat'. On entrance to the campus, near the archway he put in a dip as speed-breaker; we called it 'Thungan Fossa' borrowing an anatomical term.

The first 18 months were basic sciences. The anatomy dissection of cadavers was my favourite. Three of us planned a prank. We convinced the dissection room watchman that we were doing some late evening dissection and to leave the room open a bit late. We put a bet on with another classmate; if he could get the pen placed in the hand of a cadaver, he would get 5 rupees (which at that time would buy two decent meals). The stage was set. At about 7 PM, it was murky, also only one of the lights was switched on. The boy who agreed to take the bet went in and tried to take the pen. Suddenly, there was a loud scream. The cadaver caught hold of his hand. The 'cadaver' was one of my classmates lying still. This did not go down well with the professor and we were all reprimanded. We got away with an apology not to be silly again.

The head of general medicine was Dr Pai, an eminent physician. He was soft spoken. I might run out of adjectives to describe his qualities. He was a very analytical, balanced, caring, warm, empathetic and knowledgeable professional. On the first day of posting in medicine, he gave an introductory talk. I remember him citing Thomas Laycock. '*Each patient has a pathological as well as a mental and social individuality.*' He said, '*if you know well about diabetes you have learnt half of medicine and if you know well about syphilis, you have learnt the other half*'. Diabetes was very common at that time and syphilis was not infrequent. Both affected all systems of the body.

The wards had usually about 40 beds. But the demand was far more. Patients needing admission were admitted irrespective of bed-strength. They were given blankets and pillows to lay on the floor between beds. Sometimes a ward would have 80-90 patients.

There were lots of juvenile diabetics needing insulin. To get free treatment, they had to be formally admitted in the hospital. So these children were 'in-patients' but did not occupy beds. They used to do the shopping for essential items for the in-patients of the wards and get a small remuneration for their services. It was a symbiotic arrangement which benefitted both parties. Also to start with, the medical curriculum was tough and the audio-visual aids were in their rudimentary state. There were no computers, internet and so on. The best I had was access to the photocopier in the library which was also scarce. I went to learn typing at a Typing Institute just opposite the medical college. It was a ladies' world; owned by a lady and the full capacity of dozen students were young ladies. They started teasing me in an adorable and envious tone. "You are going to be a doctor; why do you want to learn typing?" I also started feeling like a 'fish out of water' sat among the girls in their multi-coloured sarees, hair decorated with jasmine flowers and wearing pungent perfumes. After a few weeks, I dropped out.

My grandfather's last words to me were, "Do something good every day, however trivial it is." Charity opportunities were far and few. I used to go to the blood bank and donate blood every Easter and Christmas, as a little token of my own charity. The blood bank was usually very scarce in blood. There were 'professional donors' who were crooks hanging around the blood bank extorting exorbitant amounts of money from relatives of patients in dire need of blood.

As part of the training, we had to spend two weeks at the Tuberculosis Hospital, Pulayanarkotta which was about 8 miles from the main hospital. The hospital was set in 13 acres on a hill surrounded by thick wild bushes. Due to the remoteness and proximity to peripheral jungle, rodents were frequent unwanted visitors to the wards, in search of any leftover food since many patients did not eat full meals. Snakes usually follow the trail of rodents as their main meal. So they also visited wards especially at night. Patients with various stages of Tuberculosis were in-patients there often for months to years. The World Health Organisation estimate that two-thirds of the disease is shared by eight countries, of which India had a major share. The presentation of various stages of disease was an eye-opener and a big learning experience.

After our rounds, all teams in the hospital usually went to have coffee at the Indian Coffee House just in front of the main hospital. De-brief, chit-chat, clinical discussions, gossip, current affairs, and cross reference; all matters were debated in the heatwave of coffee break.

During a summer vacation, I went to see the Taj Mahal, one of the Seven Wonders of the World. It is a white marble mausoleum on the south bank of Yamuna River, in the city of Agra, in North India. This was built on the order of Mughal Emperor Shah Jahan (reigned 1628-1658) to house the tomb of his beloved wife Mumtaz Mahal. This tourist magnet attracts 7-8 million visitors yearly. Architecture from every corner of the empire was included - Persian, Islamic, Ottoman, Turkish and Indian. Twenty-two thousand workmen and one thousand elephants worked for seventeen years to complete this marvel. The hues of the mausoleum changes from pinkish in morning, milky white in the evening and golden at night to reflect the changing moods of Mumtaz. In 1983, it was designated as UNESCO World Heritage site.

The great Mughal Emperors Akbar and Jahangir were well aware that Christianity and Islam were not far apart. They painted Jesus and Mary on palace walls. Jahangir owned a carved image of Jesus on the cross. They held courts which included representatives from all religions. Examples of mutual respect and peaceful co-existence of all religions were set in the 16th century by the great Mughal Emperors.

Taj Mahal is the ultimate jewel of Muslim art in India, which is predominantly Hindu. It is a 42 acre complex set up in formal gardens bound on three sides by crenelated battlement walls composed of a parapet with periodic rectangular indentations, to allow for a launch of arrows or other projectiles forming a defence. So many people around the world, over so many centuries tried to emulate building something similar to Taj Mahal. Only Donald Trump could do it. He built **'Trump Taj Mahal'**, a hotel and casino in Atlantic City, USA in 1990 spending just a paltry sum of US$1 billion. Alas, it did not last long; bankruptcy soon followed and it closed down in 2016. Later, it changed hands and is currently known as 'Hard Rock Hotel & Casino'.

I visited Delhi which is the capital of India. The city of Delhi actually consists of two components: Old Delhi, in the north, the historic city and New Delhi, in the south. One of the country's largest urban agglomerations, Delhi sits astride on the west bank of the Yamuna River, a tributary of the Ganges (*Ganga*) River, about 100 miles south of the Himalayas. The ridges and hillsides of the national capital territory abound in thorny trees, such as acacias, as well as seasonal herbaceous species. The sissoo tree, which yields a dark brown and durable timber, is commonly found in the plains. Riverine vegetation, consisting of weeds and grass, occurs on the banks of the Yamuna. New Delhi is known for its flowering shade trees, such as the neem, a drought-resistant tree with a pale yellow fruit, jamman tree with an edible grapelike fruit), mango and fig tree. It is also known for its flowering plants, which include a large number of multi-coloured seasonal chrysanthemums, phlox, violas, and verbenas. An upset stomach with diarrhoea by visitors, is traditionally called *Delhi Belly*.

*   *   *

During my fourth year at the medical school, one of my classmates Raj got a telegram from his close friend at home. 'Father died; Cremation next Tuesday'. He was deeply upset. His house was 35 miles away. We got him a taxi to go home straightaway. Next Tuesday, six of us went in a taxi to his house to take part in the cremation ceremony. It was a village; the taxi driver knew the area very well. We reached his house at 1.30 PM for the ceremony at 3. When we arrived, there was hardly anybody there. I said I will check over. The front door was locked. I could hear somebody talking in the backyard. So, I went around. An elderly man was lying in an easy chair in the shade of a mango tree and reading newspaper. His wife was washing clothes. I felt something spooky.

I checked, "Is this Raj's house?"

"Yes," the man replied. "Who are you?"

I replied, "I am Raj's classmate."

He said, "I am Raj's dad; he has gone to a cremation."

Soon, I got the address where Raj went. The taxi driver took us there. We put the bouquet destined for Raj's dad on the body of the deceased who was his friend's dad.

It was a stark lesson learnt in a bizarre way. Unfortunately, there were no mobile telephones then. Even landlines were 'booked calls' which would take hours before being connected.

On the way back, we visited Puthenkulam elephant village, one of the most popular tourist spots in Kollam. The place is home to more than 40 elephants, including the tallest elephant of Kerala named Puthenkulam Ananthapadmanabhan. The place is flocked by Indian as well as international visitors in great numbers, particularly during winter months (November to March). In fact, it was a great experience to spend some happy time with elephants and their mahouts carrying on with their daily life.

In the same year, one of my class mates was getting married. The wedding was 50 miles way. Due to austerity, nine of us, set out for the big day in a taxi. We were sitting stacked like sardines. The windows were open, so a few arms and heads were out in the open. The wedding was glorious. A grand meal followed. Traditionally, after meals, cigarettes and betel chewing were offered. Betel nut is the seed of the fruit of the areca palm. It is also known as areca nut. The common names, preparations and specific ingredients vary by cultural group and individuals who use it. We got back in the taxi to head back. In about 20 minutes,

I felt light-headed and nauseous. When I looked outside, I had double vision. But soon I felt a sense of well-being, euphoria, heightened alertness, sweating, salivation, a hot sensation in the body and increased vitality. In the crowded taxi three others were probably in the same boat. They all started laughing like idiots for nothing. The taxi driver got the message. He stopped near a river and asked us to get out, stretch our legs and have a nice bath in the river. He asked those of us with 'lipstick on' (betel nut chewing will turn the lips cherry red) to drink butter milk as a remedy to weaken the effects of the betel nut. The next day, most of us had a terrible headache like a sledgehammer effect and hangover feeling. Betel beats any novice with a bang. I never tried it again.

In the evenings, I used to play cricket on a regular basis. Once expelled from the Garden of Eden. Adam lost his status as a gentleman. I thought I would pick up the gentleman's game. At that time, protective equipment like helmets were far and few. The red cherry used to leave calling cards imprinted on various parts of body, sometimes giving the impression of survival after a gladiatorial fight. The college captain Dr Madan Mohan, who was also Kerala State Captain, used to say, "No pain; no gain."

When I went home, I had to convince my parents that the marks were not from picking any fights. In 1967, I went to watch the 3rd Test Match between India and the West Indies at Chepauk Stadium, Madras (now Chennai). Cricket is the opium that rejuvenates the

Indian nation. India was in a winning position at end of day 4. But the great West Indian captain Garry Sobers remained 74 not out and saved the test for them. Some people could not bear it; jumped in front of train and perished. People live and die for cricket in India and so they did.

During the fourth year, we had a four-week posting at a Primary Health Care Centre, about 50 miles away from the Medical College, at a coastal village called Neendakara, near Quilon (*Kollam*).The doctor in charge was Dr Chacko, very popular among the locals. This was the largest fishing harbour in the state. It was about 7 miles away from the city centre. Indo-Norwegian Project, Norway's first foreign aid development project, was first established in Neendakara in 1953. The aim was the modernisation of fisheries of Kerala and also improving health, sanitation and water supply. The local community was composed of mainly fishermen. We stayed there throughout the posting. An evening swim in the nearby sea was a routine fixture to wind down. Tragedy struck - a student in my junior batch drowned in the sea the following year during his placement there.

When we finished final examinations, ten of us went to Kovalam Beach to celebrate in style. We got plenty of titbits, cashew nuts, banana chips, fried chicken, chapatti, lime and mango pickles. There was an assortment of drinks - whisky, brandy and wine. Drinking lager was a taboo and considered below standard. I must emphasize that all were men since it was not considered customary or socially acceptable at those times for women to be partying with men in such a setting. Kovalam is a small coastal town south of Trivandrum. At the southern end of the beach is a striped lighthouse with a viewing platform and heading south, Vizhinjam Juma Masjid mosque overlooks the busy fishing harbour. Inland, Sagarika Marine Research Aquarium displays technology used in pearl production.

We reached our destination by 1.30 in the afternoon. There were ruined remnant seats of Halcyon castle. We spread out various food and drinks. Most of us had done the examinations well and were confident of passing. I was the Master of Ceremony. I had a football referee's whistle which I blew signalling the kick off. The celebrations kicked off in style with some spectacular fireworks. Then we all stood up, sang the national anthem in perfect harmony. Well begun is half done? All in order! Maybe the calm before the storm!

The weather goddess was very kind. There was glorious sunshine baking the occasion, it was very warm. Vibrant spells of gentle breeze from the Arabian Sea was a welcome, refreshing and stimulating accompanier. The beams of light filtering through the cascade of surrounding palm trees gave an aura of illusion with the palm tree leaves dancing in tune with the music on the ground. We took turns recalling the memorable incidents and stories spanning over five long dreaded years. Snacks...booze...stories...booze..; eating and drinking carried on, laughing, joking.

Alcohol took the lid off inhibition and self-control; singing and dancing non-stop until people were forced to take breaks to respond to calls of nature.

Everybody unwound gradually, some getting tipsy and some stumbling around. A strange couple slowly sprawled towards us, stayed and watched our antics at curiously close range. A dominant male peacock fanned his long colourful iridescent tail feathers marked with eye-like designs, followed by the peahen. The way they walked in was sending us a clear message that we are in their territory, their nocturnal halt and habitat. Maybe we were delaying their sleep.

By about 7 at night, most of us felt like winding down, tired after such hard work of eating and drinking far too much. A skylark flew into our midst interrupting the proceedings. One of my friends, who knew about birds, said it represents joy, freedom, inspiration and hope. Good omen; we were looking forward to all of these; we got it delivered. It produced a loud, sharp, mosaic of vociferous song lasting few seconds and vanished into the oblivion. I blew the whistle; the party ended. Long live our friendship.

Our graduation ceremony was at the University Hall in Trivandrum. The grand finale of five years of hard work. The degree MBBS (*Bachelor of Medicine and Bachelor of Surgery*) awarded by the university was presented by the vice-chancellor. The Dean spoke at length about the Hippocratic Oath. Hippocrates was the descendent of Aesculapius who was the son of Apollo. He had miraculous powers by which not only he cured the ill but also brought the dead back to life. This upset Zeus, the Master of The Universe since he did not want humans to be immortal and disturbing the order of the nature. So he killed Aesculapius, but being god himself, he did not vanish. He became a constellation, the serpent eater. His symbol was a snake wound around a staff. He founded a centre for healing called Epidaurus, where the rules were very stringent. In order to obtain blessings of the god, one has to have purity by fasting, abstinence and refraining sexual relations. In the dormitories where they slept, snakes visited them at night. God imparted knowledge to them in their dreams. Having taken over a heavy burden of secrecy and responsibility, I felt like a minuet of the misunderstood.

On coming out of the ceremony, we were ambushed by a barrage of choreographed high pressure marketing propaganda of specialised combat units of medical book publishers. The day came to a grinding halt by six. Like Sunday school children, as if catechism had finished, we rapidly dispersed, scattered in various packs and invaded the nearby cafés and bars in a frenzy. There was no pomp or ceremony. A few lucky people had photographs taken. After the ceremony, six of us went to Xavier's Hotel, a decent venue. We had plenty of Haywards brandy and an assortment of food which all shared at random - pappad, meat kebab, Lamb Rogan Josh, chicken tandoori, chili beef roast, paratha and rice.

By evening I got the train back home. I showed the degree rolled up in a case to my mother. She shed a few tears of joy. My father was away at work. Next day, one of my uncles who lived nearby came to see me with the newspaper which carried the report of the convocation ceremony and the list of us who received the degree. Being Abraham, my name was first. He then asked me to have a look at his knee because he had knee pain. I duly examined him. He had housemaid's knee. With a smile, he took 10 rupees and gave it to me jokingly. "Doctor, this is your private practice fee." I was reluctant to accept it but he insisted that he was giving it as a gift packed with his blessings.

5

Private Practice

'Medicine is as old as man, no doubt born of necessity and wrought by trial and error.'

Odell (2000)

Soon after graduating, I did private practice in a rural area in the high range, a village called Thalayad, a hilly rural suburb near Calicut, a prominent northern city in Kerala. The practice was busy. I had a retired pharmacist (compounder) from the army called Ajit to help me. My knowledge about the pharmacist's role was very mediocre. I encouraged him to guide me. He got an array of medicinal bottles - orange, blue, green, dark brown and clear and in various shapes.

We worked hand-in-glove as a team. I kept a dog called Jay as guard. In the night, if called upon, I used to do home visits accompanied by Ajit and Jay with torch lights and used to charge extra for the service. The locals welcomed it and I was fairly busy. One night about 10 PM, Jay barked out twice. Ajit said there may be some patient coming to see me. I was in pyjamas. I got changed and stayed in anticipation. After 10 minutes, Jay kept on barking non-stop. Since Ajit could not see anybody, he went out with the light. To our surprise it was another dog who was the potential visitor, probably on the lookout for a date with Jay. We went back to bed. I was keen to further my career by way of opportunities to work in a teaching hospital with a view to taking a post-graduate qualification.

6

Surgical Trade

'Surgeons must be very careful
When they take the knife!
Underneath their fine incisions
Stirs the Culprit—Life!'

Emily Dickinson

After about eight months, I closed the clinic and joined
Calicut Medical College. I was a tutor under Associate
Professor BT Nayar FRCS. He was one of the finest
surgeons I have come into contact with. When I met
him first, I got the impression that he was a true
gentleman. Edmund Burke commented, '*A king may
make a nobleman but he cannot make a gentleman*'. It is true,
gentlemen are self-made. He set examples in thought,
word and deed. He was always on time. If anybody was
late, the latecomer has to sign the attendance register in
red. Moreover, two reds would end up meeting the
cost of coffee and snacks of our weekly meeting. He
was an excellent surgeon and continued to stimulate
lateral thinking. He used to mentor and shape the
qualities befitting a surgeon. He had an eagle's eye and

lion's heart. He encouraged me to take a post-graduate qualification by saying, "You must put knife before wife" meaning to take a Master's Degree before getting married. There was a placard hanging on his wall which read:

'To study the phenomenon of disease without books is to sail uncharted sea, while to study books without patients is not to go to sea at all.'

Sir William Osler [1849-1919]

He used to have journal club weekly. All of us had to bring up something new which has cropped up in recent journals. I found that to be the best pragmatic stimulus of continuous learning and improvement all my life. Dr Nayar had high expectations from all subordinate staff. I pay my great tribute to him for all the training and guidance.

I was staying in hospital quarters at a subsidised rate. Work was hectic. I used to play cricket and tennis on an irregularly regular basis. For company, I brought a Bonnet Macaque monkey. I named him Sen. He was my constant companion. I got him well trained. He would bring me the post, pick up the telephone when it rang and howl at any strangers coming to the door unless I signalled him to stop. Also, if I didn't give him much needed attention, he would sit on my lap and look at me almost asking 'What is the matter'? He would eat with me sat on his adapted chair. Although I had made a bed especially for him, he would come into my bedroom often. So, I moved his bed into my bedroom so that both of us felt the company better. Later on, it was reported in the press, Shipar Reza in Bangladesh had a dog called Mintu who became a surrogate mother feeding an orphaned monkey, who also rode on her back.

The population explosion was a problem looming in India. The government was actively seeking measures. The Sunday schools were converted to vasectomy camps. Myself and colleagues, usually half a dozen doctors, would start the camp about 9 in the morning and work till 6 in the evening. About 400-500 men would be queuing up. They were led into a registration room where basic administration was done, next was the preparation room where they were shaved and briefed, then they came into the doctor's room. The vasectomy was done under local anaesthetic and took about 20 minutes. After the procedure, the man would get a bucket full of rice and vegetables, a pair of clothes and 25 rupees. It was quite an incentive at those times. I used to get paid the paltry sum of 3 rupees per patient. We did it more as a service to the nation and the profession rather than on pecuniary interest.

One evening, while on duty, I got a call from the Casualty department. A 35 year-old lady had been left abandoned at the door after being knocked down by a car and she was dying. I rushed in. The house officer had put a drip on her. The lady was in the ragged clothes of labourer and appeared with deathly pallor. A quick examination confirmed she was in shock. I arranged for her to be taken to theatre for an immediate operation. On the way, I went to the blood bank to get blood for her. There was no blood available. I asked the technician to bleed me and took my blood with me and ran to theatre. On opening her abdomen, there was blood all over. She had a ruptured spleen. I operated while my blood was being given and was able to stabilise her. She made a wonderful recovery and was discharged home after seven days. She beat everybody - the reckless car driver, nature, science and medicine. Indeed she did!

I used to attend to lots of assault and traffic accident cases, which used to end up in courts. The cases would come up before the courts about eight months to a year after. As the doctor who treated, I would be summoned to court as an expert witness. About three or four days a month, I had to go to courts often in remote areas far away. Although it was bit of a challenging experience, I used to enjoy it because of the travel, break from routine and meeting new people. Doctors were generally well respected in the courts. Once I ended up in a court about 70 miles away. Only when I got into the witness box, I realised that the magistrate was my uncle. We both didn't know until I got in the court. It was a pleasant surprise. Also, I got a free meal after the hearing.

About 80 miles south of Calicut, is the vibrant City of Thrissur, 'the cultural capital of Kerala'. Thrissur Pooram is an annual Hindu festival held in May. People celebrate the festival crossing all barriers of religion, caste and community. The celebration is a spectacle that has amazed and delighted people for the past three centuries. Tens of thousands of people take part and the festival always has a complement of enthusiastic foreign tourists. The firecrackers, the special delicacies, the decorations and most importantly the majestic elephants are all a lifetime experience. This festival has been an inspiration for so many other festivals within Kerala and outside. It is a seven day festival starting with the flag hoisting ceremony (*Kodiyettam*). This is followed, on the fourth day, by the sample firecrackers ceremony. Many colourful displays of firecrackers are the norm and the atmosphere is almost frenzied. Everybody prepares excitedly for the main day.

The main *Pooram* (on the sixth day) happens every year on the day when the *Pooram* star rises in the sky in the Malayalam month of *Medam*. The Raja and the priests of the two other important local temples, the *Paramekkavu Bagavathi* Temple and the *Thiruvambadi Sri Krishna* Temple, pay obeisance to Shiva, the presiding deity of the *Vadakkunnathan* Temple. To this day the priests of the other two temples and their processions stand opposite each other and celebrate Lord Shiva whose idol is placed in the centre. These two temples compete with and try to outwit each other in the procession. They bring fifteen elephants, each decorated to dazzle. All the ornaments are hand-crafted by artisans who are specially called to work at the temple premises. The accoutrements are added with great attention to detail.

The spectators too catch the fever of the tournament-like ambience. Both sides alternately exchange colourful umbrellas and fans in perfect rhythm and every time this happens there are cheers from the onlookers. All this, while the musical combination of *nadaswarams* and drums beat away, enhance the effect of the spectacle. On the seventh day there is again a fantastic display of firework at the Swaraj ground, a fitting finale to the almost electric revels of the preceding days.

After three years of intense studies and training, I passed Master of Surgery (M.S) from Kottayam Medical College in central Kerala. My batch mate from medical school, Dr Mathew, was doing private practice in a nearby village. He started his medical curriculum in Germany; so he was called *German Mathew*. We used to meet quite often. He was the kindest man I have ever met. He had pleasant manners, amicable predisposition and an infectious smile which would linger on forever.

Although his practice was private, he would treat the poor patients often free of charge, a rare quality among aspiring doctors who want to establish themselves and build up a decent bank balance. Patients liked him so much that he got invited to every ceremony in the village - baptisms, weddings and other celebrations. Unfortunately, he developed persistent cough, later diagnosed as lung cancer and he died a premature death.

'Many people will walk in and out of your life, but only true friends will leave footprints in your heart'- Eleanor Roosevelt.

Indeed, Mathew has left many footprints in my heart. RIP my friend.

7

African Sojourn

'The world is a book, and those who do not travel read only a page.'

St Augustine

I saw an advertisement in *The Indian Express* newspaper requesting job applications for the post of surgeon in Ethiopia with quite attractive terms – a salary five times more than I was getting, free air ticket, 4 weeks annual leave and free accommodation. I sent the application. In two weeks, I was called for interview in Madras. On the third day, I got the telegram telling me that I had been successful. In another three weeks, I finalised my trip to Ethiopia. I flew from Cochin to Bombay. I had to stay overnight at Hotel Centaur, a 5-star hotel in Bombay before catching a flight to Addis Ababa next day. After living in a frugal way in hospital quarters, sudden sight of enormous luxury and comfort in a 5-star hotel where many celebrities have stayed, brought on goose pimples due to sheer excitement.

The room was on the 7th floor, with a sit-out terrace overlooking the Arabian Sea. It had a high ceiling, mahogany furniture, leather chairs and a king-sized bed. The en-suite bathroom had a shower and free-standing Victoria bath. There was a central ornate chandelier with discrete up-lights in all four corners. A mini bar with a glass decanter attracted my special attention. The bathroom had a central sculptural pendant lamp in the middle along with various concealed lights creating a sense of subtle glow and intimacy. The layout was a testament and relic of the timeless elegance of the British Raj.

The phone rang a few minutes later. The caller said he was the personal butler and sought my permission to come in. I let him in. He gave a vivid overview of his CV having served many Hollywood stars and international statesman. He had a photo album to prove his credentials of meeting these VIPs. He used flattery saying that, "One day you will be among these names." He gave a picturesque and mouth-watering description of the various gourmet meals he could make for me. Concealing my diffidence and ignorance in this unchartered territory, I replied, "I am too tired, I want to take some rest. I shall get back to you later if needed." He said I could ring him on his extension or I could go to the restaurant any time and there was plenty to choose from.

Later, I went to the restaurant. The dinner was the first proper one I enjoyed in my life because it was sumptuous, of 5-star quality and most importantly complementary with air travel. It started with Dom Perignon champagne served in a coupe. I had seen champagne flutes before, but it was the first time I saw a coupe. The coupe was modelled on the left breast of Queen Marie Antoinette, wife of King Louis XVI of France. Although I had tasted champagne once before, this was the opportunity to drink it to my satisfaction without any inhibitions whatsoever. I seized the moment with both hands. It tasted of combined delicacy, subtle freshness and skilful blending. It was pure and toned with incredible balance between nose and palate. I filled coupe after coupe until I started seeing shining stars.

My starter was Tuna Tartar Cocktail with avocado and cucumber relish. My salivary system went into overdrive. Sorbet, oven-roasted oysters with garlic butter, parsley, chives and mushrooms. Main dish was pot-roasted venison with port, cranberries and chestnut gravy. Moroccan pistachio rice, sweet potato and mixed leaf salad were plenty to go with. There were half a dozen desserts which I could not fathom out and by that time I was too full. So I was content with fruit salad. I was so tired after the heaviest meal in my life, felt like a python who had a heavy prey and went to bed shortly.

Next morning about 7.30, the phone rang to say that the flight has been postponed to the next day due to a technical problem with the aircraft. I decided to have an overview of Bombay. Mumbai (formerly called Bombay) is a densely populated city on India's west coast. A financial centre, it's India's largest city. On the Mumbai Harbour waterfront stands the iconic Gateway of India stone arch, built by the British Raj in 1924. Offshore, nearby Elephants Island holds ancient cave temples dedicated to the Hindu god Shiva. The city's also famous as the heart of the Bollywood film industry.

Bombay Architecture came to be present through the British in the 18th and early 19th centuries. At first it was the neoclassical style of architecture but later, the Victorian Gothic style came to dominate the city. Where the neoclassical has an orderly monochromatic presence, the Gothic style is expressive, disjointed with surfaces of lives colours, beautified with carved and narrative elements, consisting of flying buttresses, lancet windows and stained glass. At first, due to the immense freed space it obtained, Gothic buildings only served as churches, as religious buildings built by people of the 11th century. However, soon enough there came a need for public halls, parliament houses, mansions, and the Gothic era was the solution. Indian architects came to analyse this style and represent it and put it into play in relation with the climate, and in relation to society's plans and sensibilities. This style, the blend of Gothic and contemporary styles, is what came to be known as 'Bombay Gothic.'

According to writer Jan Morris, "Bombay is one of the most characteristically Victorian cities in the world, displaying all the grand effrontery of Victorian eclecticism." The British influence on buildings in the city is evident from the colonial era. However, the architectural features include a range of European influences such as German gables, Dutch roofs, Swiss timbering, Romance arches and Tudor casements often fused with traditional Indian features.·

Many Bollywood stars live in Mumbai. Also it is the home of the 'God of Cricket', Sachin Tendulakar. One-time richest man in the world, Mukesh Ambani lives in a house 60-storeys tall with his wife and three children. But there is an Indian living in the north-eastern state of Mizoram called Ziona Chana who lives in a modest 4 storied building with 100 rooms, with 39 wives, 94 children and 33 grandchildren- all under one roof. He must be the greatest diplomat on earth!

*　　　　　　　*　　　　　　　*

The next day, my flight departed as scheduled. My first international flight. I braced myself with aspirations and inspirations for the future lying ahead. The flight landed in Addis Ababa around 4.30 PM. It was winter time with a chilling temperature of two degrees Celsius. It was murky. I got a taxi to the hotel eight miles away. While lazily glancing I noticed a dead body lying on side of the road. I thought it was cattle. When I asked, the driver said that the military now let bodies lie for a day or two after overnight shooting to teach a lesson to anybody who opposes the regime. A sudden chill went down my spine. I had a dry mouth and words were not coming out due to fear and anxiety. The driver was kind and considerate. He tried to reassure me that I would get a special pass being a doctor and the military usually like foreign doctors.

I reached the Plaza hotel in Piazza square. With jet lag and exhaustion due to fear of the unknown, I went to bed about 9 PM after two shots of whisky and a heavy meal. Soon I slipped into a state of narcosis. About 2 AM, I was woken up by gun shots at very close range. Terrified, I got up and opened the window to see what is going on. I could not find any activities outside. I pulled the mattress down onto floor and laid down thinking that even if the gunshot came at window level, I would be safe. Quarter of an hour later, I heard some thumping noise of thuds approaching. There were two loud knocks with heavy metal on my door. I hesitated to open. Then there was a loud order to open the door. On opening, two soldiers with rifles and attached bayonets were pointing at me and shouted something in Aramaic (local language). I was shivering like a leaf and raised both hands above my shoulder level. The hotel duty manager was with them. On enquiry, the soldiers thought I was giving some signals out on hearing the gun shots. The manager explained that I am the new doctor at the hospital, they smiled and left with a warning not to put light on or open the window if I hear gunshots. So the first night was one of terror and drama.

Next morning I went to the Black Lion Hospital and met Dr Bhatt, the Chief Surgeon. He was five feet eight inches tall, athletic build, with pale complexion, gleaming black hair and thick black eyebrows. With a warm welcoming smile, he shook hands and introduced me to another doctor in his room who was a physician. He took me to the administration office to complete various formalities and accommodation. The administrator said that the military would impose curfews as and when and be mindful when going out of hospital campus. She said to display the hospital pass at all times and if any military personnel asks anything, first raise both hands straight up over the shoulders. After finishing the introductory rituals, we sat to have a coffee with Dr Bhatt. He went through my surgical experience. I had already brought from India a set of general surgery instruments. He appeared very pleased with me.

The work routine was very hectic - weekly two operation days and two nights duty. I enjoyed being busy at work. Life after work was very dragging, no friends and social life. I started feeling lonely. Also the unexpected curfews started hurting me. After work, I used to go around sight-seeing. St George's cathedral is one of the finest churches I have visited. St George is the patron saint of Ethiopia. Emperor Menelik II built to commemorate his defeat of the Italians. It has distinctive octagonal form in neoclassical style with grey stone exterior. The interior is studded with ornate paintings and mosaics. Adjacent to the cathedral, there is a museum with a collection of ecclesiastical paraphernalia- crowns, holy scrolls, ceremonial umbrellas, coronation grabs of Emperors Zewdith and

Haile Selassie. Mount Entoto is the highest peak about 3000 metres above mean sea level. It was always chilly. Emperor Menelik II built his palace there. It is densely populated with eucalyptus trees and called 'the lung of Addis Ababa'.

My love of monkeys led me to visit Beehner's camp in the Simien Mountain National Park. That was home to the Gelada monkeys, who are exotic and socially adventurous primates. They have striking burning eyes and leathery complexions. It is estimated that about 100,000 live there. Males are the size of large dogs and females usually half the male's size. They do falsetto cries, barks and grunts depending on the situation. Males frequently display their canines like those of vampires as a show of strength. Both sexes are bald. An hour-glass patch of skin on their chest broadcasts male's social status and female's reproductive state.

They move about in herds. Each herd is led by a male and up to a dozen females in his harem along with the offspring. They mainly feed on grass. Cows and sheep compete with them for the grass. In the night, they sleep on the edges of cliffs on ledges out of grasp of predators like leopards and hyenas. The life of the monarch is in danger as he gets older. Potential young stronger bachelors threaten him. Sometimes gladiatorial battles evolve with biting, hair pulling and scratching. If the leader is deposed, he is demoted in the harem to look after the young in an avuncular role but most importantly he loses his mating rights.

On Sundays, I used to go to church. In the church, I
met Mike, a Nigerian. He was very friendly and
knowledgeable. We became friends and used to meet
weekly. A few weeks later, he said he was going to
Nigeria for three weeks. Mike contacted me when he
came back. He told me that they were looking for
surgeon at Ife University, which is the area he hails
from. He gave me the contact details. I corresponded
with the university and I was offered a job there. After
giving notice to the employer and serving eight
months, I left Addis and landed in Lagos.

8

Mission Nigeria

'Every part of Nigeria is blessed.'

Ifeanyi Onuoha

I got the job as surgical registrar in Ife University. It
was a much hotter climate than Ethiopia. On the third
day, after my evening meal, I felt light-headed and
feverish. I went to bed about 9.30 PM. By 11, I started
vomiting and could not function at all. There was no
phone in the quarters. I managed to walk to one of the
nearby hospital wards. The nurse, Kim, was sat up
writing some notes. She appeared to be about 25, with
child-like eyes, dark lush hair and a thin beautiful
mouth curving to produce a radiant smile. There was a
sense of high voltage about her. With an affected
assumption of fear and doubt I briefly explained to her
how I felt. She pondered while gazing at me and
displayed an encouraging sentiment. Her instant
remark was, "Are you the new surgeon?"

I said, "Yes."

With a sympathetic smile, she said, "Doctor, you have got malaria. You may go back to the quarters. I will come in about 15 minutes." Although I was astonished and bewildered by her spot diagnosis, I felt reassured that she would be right.

Leaving the door open, I laid flat on the sofa, exhausted and awaiting my fate. A short while later the door was noiselessly opened and Kim breezed into the room and asked me to turn over. In no time, she gave me an injection on my buttocks - Nivaquin. Then she gave me paracetamol tablets. I nodded in the direction of the chair inviting her to sit down. She sat for two minutes, checked my temperature and pulse and left before I could even say thanks. I nodded off in partial state of delirium. About 4 in the morning, Kim came with some coffee and toast and woke me up. I had been sweating profusely and on waking up felt like a big weight has been offloaded from my head. I felt that I got the best coffee which rejuvenated my inner self. By 7 in the morning, I took the follow up tablets and rested. By tea time, I was almost 80% back to normal. I was fine and well in three days. I felt I had crossed the first hurdle of the new chapter in my life.

Every minute, a child in Africa still dies from malaria. Malaria is most common in poor, deprived areas. In many cases, malaria itself is the cause of such poverty: malaria causes havoc on a socioeconomic level as patients are often bedridden and incapable of carrying out normal daily tasks, resulting in burdens on households and health services, and ultimately huge losses to income in malaria-endemic countries. This suffering and loss of life are tragically unnecessary because malaria is largely preventable, detectable and treatable.

I was posted to Wesley Guild Hospital, Ilesha, annexe of Ife University. The chief surgeon was Michael who had postgraduate training from America. Very soon, we got to know each other. He was pleased with my surgical skills and gave me a free hand. I did my best to relieve as much pressure off him. On a weekend I had to operate on about twenty-five emergencies - appendectomy, obstructed hernia, perforated stomach ulcers, stab injuries, other accidents, head injuries etc. The demand was very challenging and gave me a great deal of experience.

I was put up in the hospital quarters. There was a caretaker lady called Esther. She did cleaning, tidying and essential cooking as needed. She used to come with her 8 month-old son Lawrence tied firmly on her back. I noticed that he was not active and suffered from severe malnutrition called marasmus. I told Esther to feel free to give him plenty to eat and drink with special emphasis on milk and make use of items in the fridge. Almost, in a week I could see he started thriving. In the following three months, he reached his normal weight and started walking.

The Ilesha community was small, warm and friendly. Most importantly, people got to know me as patients and became friends. Many items like beer were scarce to buy in the open market. There were certain shops where they hiked the price. Being the doctor, I got them at recommended price and at times as complements, small perks attached to the job. Saturday markets were very popular and bustling. All sorts of meat - chicken, beef, sheep, dog, bush meat (rat) and snakes - were on show to pick and choose from.

One day, at the outpatients, I got a note from a doctor from neighbouring village who referred an 83 year-old man called Jacob for a hernia operation. He appeared to be only 55. When I enquired about his daily routine he said he had to ferry his 15 grandchildren to school which was 2 miles way as 3 trips of 5 children placed in front and back on his bike morning and evening. In between he would do household errands like going to market, fetching water etc. He did not have a trace of fat on his body. No wonder he looked that young and healthy.

I also got to know Joshua who was a senior car dealer. He invited me to his 55th birthday party. There were about a hundred people there. Plenty of food and drinks were at our disposal. There were chicken, beef, bush meat (rat) and fish. Halfway through, he was going around meeting all the guests. When he came to me, he noticed I was holding a near-empty plate. Joshua remarked, "I am very pleased. Some of you (foreigners) want to pass through the country but they don't want the country to pass through them."

About 15 miles away, there was a natural waterfall with warm water at a place called Ikogosi. Over some weekends, I used to go down and have a dip in the warm spring.

After a monotonous day's work, I was on call for the night. About six in the evening, the hospital manager contacted me to say that the duty obstetrician was involved in an accident and was hospitalised and requested me to hold the fort until another doctor could be drafted in to replace him. Although I had reasonable experience in handling most surgical problems, my obstetric skills were rusty. Reluctantly I agreed to cover the interim time.

Almost half an hour later, I got a call from the Casualty Department that a lady had been brought in with labour pains. As I was heading towards her the corridor echoed her loud screams; she was in real pain. On the end-on view, I could not see her face; just only a massively protuberant abdomen which was blocking her face. My first impression was that she had twins. She hailed from a nearby village and was destined for a home labour. Only when things got out of control, the family decided to bring her to hospital. There was no facility to scan. I examined her thoroughly. Meanwhile she desperately wanted to go to toilet. On return, I examined her - to my horror the membranes had ruptured, the cord was prolapsing. This was absolute indication for an immediate Caesarean section. The anaesthetist was living eight miles way; to get him I had to send a request with an ambulance. There was no blood available in the blood bank.

If I did not operate immediately, not only the babies but also the mother would die. The nearest hospital with better facilities was fifteen miles away - about half an hour journey. There was every possibility that she might die if I were to send her there. To operate without an anaesthetist and blood might result in death on the table.

Caught between Scylla and Carbides, I had no one to turn to. I knelt in the side-room, buried my face in my hands and prayed. "Oh God…please give me the courage and skill to tackle the situation; please help me to bring the babies safely into the world and take care of the mother." I looked around for some form of refuge. The words of the professor on the first day in medical school rang in my ears. "Don't hesitate to cut your stethoscope to use as airway if somebody is choking; don't waver; act straightaway."
Procrastination is the thief of time. I felt the moment had come; the moment to act. I remembered the song in my choir-boy days 'Lead, Kindly Light amid the encircling gloom, Lead thou me on'.

There was a sudden gush of blood as my head pumped up with surge of adrenaline. I called the nurse, the ward orderly, the patient and husband; explained the utmost gravity of the situation and my decision to do a caesarean operation under local anaesthetic. All were in full agreement. Another look at the patient - she clutched my hands and said, "Help me; God will reward you." I took a deep breath and looked at her and her husband with an immense sense of conviction and devotion.

Another nurse was called in to observe the patient. I started a drip. After preparation, I gave local anaesthetic and started the operation. On the first cut, the blood sprayed onto the theatre light producing a starry sky effect. My heart was pounding with a complex myriad of emotions - fear, apprehension and emotional turbulence. If the worst happens, will I be struck off or prosecuted? The joke from medical school days wandered into my mind: 'the operation was a success but the patient died'. Soon the thoughts melted way and I was filled with excitement.

My concentration reached the pinnacle. The operation went according to plan. When I took the first baby out, it didn't cry. The nurse gave a tap and there was a loud cry - a bouncing boy. The loud scream of joy from the mother reverberated from the theatre to the next room and echoed back. Soon followed the second - a baby girl. Both were fine. I noticed every flicker of the mother's eyebrows in the serene theatre light. Due to heavy bleeding, I applied lots of clamps and started closing the abdomen. Everything went smooth. I got out and thanked God.

The entire clan of the couple arrived at the hospital and were eagerly waiting like the multitude anxious to see the white smoke of the Sistine Chapel during the Conclave. The retinue had flocked into the hospital ground. The news of the births was greeted with a thunder of joy - laughing, screaming, shouting and drinking. The cacophony of voices singing my praise was astounding. Conscious of the fact that I was the centre of attention, I peered around with a broad smile and remarked, "I only started the operation; the guardian angel was looking over me and guided me to completion." I was reminded of the 16th century French barber surgeon Ambroise Pare's words - *'Je le pansai, Dieu le guerit '* (I dressed him, and God healed him).

Like a sorcerer who has performed a miracle, I went to my living quarters. Soon the sheer catharsis of emotions led to a state of euphoria which transformed into slumber. The mother and babies were fine. They were discharged on the tenth day as planned. A great sense of pride and satisfaction permeated the air on their discharge. The couple with the new arrivals visited me. They brought a crate of beer, a hen and two chicks symbolising mother and babies. I brought up the hen and chicks until I left Nigeria when I gave them as a parting gift to a friend of mine. 'Being a hero is the shortest-lived profession on earth.'

*   *   *

I went on holiday to India for a month. The flight from Lagos to Bombay was a night flight. Although I was in the non-smoking area, the seat I got was just behind the smoking section. I noticed a young lady had been chain-smoking and drinking wine glass after glass.

A couple of hours later, I got a burnt smell, to my horror, she had been asleep and a cigarette stub from the overfull ash tray, slipped on the floor. I alerted the air hostess, who ran in and quickly extinguished the fire. I cited this incident and wrote to International Air Traffic Authority that all flights should be non-smoking. It took many years before that became a reality.

One day, when I came back from work, there was a letter which read, 'Next Tuesday, we will be visiting your street. Please leave the car key on ignition. Do not inform the police. If so, you will be in danger'. I checked with my neighbour Joe who confirmed it is from an armed robbery gang. He said, "A murderous-looking man with a square wooden face came riding on a bike and dropped that letter in your letter box."

I froze for a few moments, my eyes drooped and I sat down, elbows resting on the table, lowered my face in my hands. My mind was travelling like a bullet train, with heart pounding and sweating. After being in the same position for twenty minutes, I got some far-fetched mental strength and made up my mind to leave the country. In December 1983, we left Nigeria and flew into the UK.

9

Passage to Britain

'England has been called, with great felicity of conception, "the land of liberty and good sense". We have preserved many of the advantages of a free people, which the nations of the Continent have long since lost.'

William Godwin

1984 was a leap year, which read 5744-45 on the Hebrew Calendar. That year, Prince Harry was born, Steve Redgrave won the first of his five Olympic gold medals. The song *Do they know it's Christmas?* was released. I started work in the NHS. My first job was at C&A Hospital, Bangor in the surgical department as a Senior House Officer. At that time, most staff spoke in Welsh to each other and to patients. So I felt like a fish out of water. Then they would try to talk in English as well. I worked there for nearly four weeks. The consultant surgeon Mr Roberts was very caring, supportive and helpful. He guided me to get the next job.

I moved to Abergavenny to work at Neville Hall Hospital. The market town was very picturesque with a warm and lovely population. There were about two dozen Asian faces in the town, most of whom were doctors. Work was in the accident and emergency department. It was quite busy and got hectic in summer time. Some days, the queue of patients was so long and waiting times of many hours.

*   *   *

I got a job at Halifax Royal Infirmary. So, we moved to a house at Sowerby Bridge. The town was originally a fording point over the once much-wider River Calder where it joins the River Ryburn. The town takes its name from the historic bridge which spans the river in the town centre. The textiles and engineering industry grew up around the bridge. By the mid-19th century the population had grown and the settlement became an urban district in the West Riding of Yorkshire in 1894. From 1892 to 1930 Pollit & Wigzell manufactured stationary steam engines for the cotton and woollen mills of Yorkshire, Lancashire and India. Wood Brothers, an engineering and millwright company, also produced engines from its Valley Iron Works. The Markfield Beam Engine in north London is an example of its work.

My wife Mary used to collect children from school and go to a shop in Sowerby Bridge owned by Stan and

Lynn Overend. Stan was an ex-airman with the RAF
marine branch and served in India, Sri Lanka and
Singapore during World War II. Lynn worked as an
ATS lady along with Stan. He used to keep them
entertained by narrating his days in the Far East with
pleasure and poise of nostalgia. They moved to
Seaburn in Sunderland. We kept in touch all the time
and we have visited them off and on. He lived in a
quiet cul-de-sac. His 1952 black Morris Minor was
parked in the take-off position. He used to narrate his
experiences of war which were reflective of his
inventiveness, ingenuity and adaptation to extreme
hostile and alien conditions. By a lottery grant from the
Help for Heroes Support Scheme, both Stan and Lynn
went to Sri Lanka to re-live the memories of their past.
Stan died aged 94 in March 2018 after a brief illness.
RIP, my friend.

With a view to get into general practice, I took
professional advice. I needed to do at least six months
in a medical specialty. Psychiatry was the prudent
choice since almost half the GP consultations have
some underlying mental health issues. Also, it was
much easier to get the job than acute medicine. I did
psychiatry at Bolton Hospital. It was a very busy but
rewarding and enterprising experience. In the third
week at about 2.30am and while on duty, I was called
from Accident and Emergency Department to attend
to a young man (24), while male. He was brought by
his neighbour in a disturbed state and staff said he was
potentially violent. I went into the cubicle and greeted
him, "Good morning." He had a quick look at me and

shouted, "I don't want a Paki doctor to see me."
Although I felt embarrassed momentarily, regaining
composure, I replied, "I am here to help you as the
duty doctor. Can you tell me what is bothering you?"
He then turned away and curled into a foetal position,
shouted, "f…, go away,"… and covered his head with
the blanket. I asked for assistance from the nurse. She
tried to persuade him to talk to me but it was all in
vain. I spoke to the consultant who came down and
assessed him. He was not willing for any treatment or
admission. He was sectioned under the Mental Health
Act and was admitted to the ward. Two days later,
when I saw him in the ward, he was very friendly and
apologised to me for his outburst at the onset.

That was the first time, somebody has behaved in an
overtly racist manner to me. I cite the comments of a
prominent GP, Dr Dipak Ray (*Migrant Architects of the
NHS* by Julian Simpson, p.128) about a colleague at a
medical meeting: '*The guy came, was cracking jokes
about…..OHMS [On Her Majesty's Service]. There's so many
bloody foreigners, he said, actually OHMS is 'Only Hindus,
Muslims and Sikhs'…* Dr Ray challenged him. '*I am going
to take it up with the Secretary of State'*. Although I have
felt occasional overtures of hidden racism in hospital
practice, it has never bothered me. I believe that if we
change the angle we look at things, things will change
in our direction although it might take its own time. I
have found the other side of the coin. After being in
general practice for a while, on many occasions patients
have come to me to double check whether the

medication changes done in the hospital by born and bred English consultants, are acceptable.

10

Plunge into General Practice

'It cannot be too often or too forcibly brought home to us that the hope of the profession is with the men who do its daily work in general practice.'

William Osler

After working in various hospitals, I felt I was being controlled by quixotic dictators - men in grey suits, who controlled every nanosecond of my career. Patients often gave the impression that they were in a transit lounge. Often they remarked, "When I get back, I will sort it out with my doctor (GP)." Winston Churchill's physician Lord Moran's words were in my ears. *'GPs were the unfortunates who have fallen off the ladder of professional development.'* I decided to take up general practice because I felt my career progress had been ossified, I could not lead a nomadic lifestyle of moving to a new job every six months and my children moving to new schools so often.

We moved from Bolton to Beverley, close to the Beverley Minster, a masterpiece of Gothic architecture. Although the construction started in 1190, the progress was slow with various interruptions like the *Black Death* and reached completion by late 15th century. It is worth mentioning the minister at Beverley Minster, Reverend Joseph Coltman, who held his role from 1823 to 1844. He held the record of being the heaviest man in England for a length of time, weighing 37st 8lbs. To propel himself around, he had a 'dandy-horse' velocipede, a modified bicycle. He was a very kind and benevolent man and died at 60. I was reminded of Sydney Smith's words about his brother. 'He has risen by his gravity and I have been sunk by my levity.'

In 1992, Presidents Bush and Yelstin proclaimed the end of Cold War; the queen celebrated her ruby jubilee. In the same year, as a humble mortal, I started as a partner in general practice in Bransholme in Hull. It was one of Europe's biggest council estates. The phenomenal problems encountered while training there, fuelled my aspiration to confront them.

The practice had four partners with over 7000 patients located in two surgeries at north and south. The surgery had a full complement of staff - practice manager, secretary, five receptionists, three nurses and attached health visitors, district nurses and physiotherapist. There were three bouts of vandalism in two years, latest resulting in 64 smashed skylights.

Morning surgery was usually 35 to 40 patients, followed by 3 to 4 home visits. I had to do lots of administration and paperwork in the afternoon. Evening surgery composed of 25-30 patients. During the week, antenatal clinics, child health clinics and minor surgery were interspersed.

The receptionists formed the bridge. They were pleasant, well-dressed, smiling, caring and helpful to patients and others. Theirs is probably the most stressful job in the health service. The receptionist is the glass prism through which the patient sees the image of the doctor. A problem can be half-solved by a skilled receptionist. A daily dose of one gram of praise and a teaspoon of nice words from the doctor is the ideal tonic to get them going. Although not politically trained they were excellent in public relations. The phone never stopped - they had to deal with an avalanche of urgent calls, dozens of patients wanting to speak to doctor, social services, coroner, pharmacists etc. My key message to them was simple, "Be brief but not abrupt." Some patients were so rude that it would have made Alexander Graham Bell turn in his grave to see the blatant abuse of his creation.

The secretary did a wonderful job. She worked in a crowded office with phones ringing around her. She did all the typing of letters to and from hospital, social services, insurance companies, solicitors and what not. She was an expert in reading 'doctor's handwriting' and better than the chemists. She was one of the best staff I have worked with in my career. The ever glowing smile was her landmark with her patent on it. In 1995, I wrote an article called '2020 Vision', how general practice will be in 2020 for the magazine, *DOCTOR*. It came runner-up in a national competition. It was more her typing than my writing which got me that accolade. I express my gratitude to her. She left this world prematurely due to illness. I pay my great tribute to you, Denise, from the bottom of my heart. Rest in peace!

Most house visits were for the elderly. Opportunistic visits while visiting somebody in the area were rewarding since they felt wanted and gave the impression that the doctor was caring. Running child health clinics was an important job. The mothers enjoyed regular weighing. Undressing before weighing was useful to pick up skin rashes, non-accidental injuries etc.

Sir Archibald Garrod commented, 'Individual cases of any particular disease, infective or other, are not exactly alike, as are the prints pulled out from a lithographic block; they resemble rather the drawings made from the same model by individual members of a drawing class. Although the differences may be slight, one has to be careful in interpretation of the case scenario.'

One of my favourite patients whom I spent a lot of time with, was a 10 year-old boy. He underwent a rare operation for bile duct obstruction - Kasai operation and liver transplant. The post-operative period was stormy with respiratory distress and sepsis. He had recurrent bowel disturbances and was on immunosuppressive therapy. He was blessed with marvellous parents who enjoyed every moment of his life in sickness and health.

The first thing that strikes anybody who visited this area, is the bewildering way in which the houses are numbered. It was regularly irregular. Ambulance staff, midwives and other health professionals were among those who got lost. It was like driving on the continent - everything seemed the wrong way around. Unemployment, crime, drug abuse and almost all facets of anti-social activities were manifested. Car burning at times was a hobby. Street lights were shattered to aid and abet nocturnal activities.

Some patients asked for home visits frequently and for trivial matters. Like the US President's plane 'Air force One', my car had to be equipped to deal with all problems - be they medical, domestic or social. Problems with neighbours, vandalism, theft and requests to sign social security papers were all reasons to demand home visits. Many expected a rapid response after requesting home visit with threats to call an ambulance if doctor did not come quickly. Also, there was a strange malady of *surgery phobia*. Some would ring and make appointment at surgery but make every effort not to attend. We tried to educate the masses with not much success.

Most people are reluctant to discuss or expose the details of their home life to benevolent strangers. One of the main problems of life in a council estate is overcrowding. Although they start as a couple or small family, in a short span of time they have two or four children. In a confined space they endure childbirth, sickness and domestic quarrels. These lead to slovenly and untidy ways, culinary slackness and a generalised easy-going approach to day to day life. Unemployment and yolk of financial worries compound the issues. I am not a saint to judge the matters. Most people in that situation might act in similar ways. This has been a national scandal over decades. The governments of the time have been building more houses and various charities have been pulling their weight to address the problems. The NHS does not charge a fee for restoring somebody's health or saving a life. The society has to adapt and change the attitude to restore health, self-respect and pride of the individuals who are less lucky and lagging behind.

One night about 1 AM, I got a call from a 62 year-old lady who was feeling sick and giddy. She was calling from her daughter's house; I spoke to the daughter and promised to visit her there. About an hour later, daughter rang me checking how much longer it would take for me to get there. I told her I am just ten minutes away and asked her to put on the outside light and be on the lookout for me. As usual, the street lights were not working. I drove slowly trying to locate the house.

Suddenly, a woman approached my car and I stopped. As I asked her how her mother was, she got into my car. The vivid prospect of my name appearing in the local press for 'kerb crawling' filled me with panic. I ran with my case to the nearest house with lights on. It was a taxi driver who pointed me to the right house. But he helped to chase the woman away while I attended to the patient. After that encounter, I always put central locking on while travelling at night.

Putting the horror stories aside, the vast majority of patients were friendly and upheld traditional values. Their affection and warmth kept me going. As a GP, I had the unique opportunity to see through the stark realities that lie beneath the social surface of fellow human beings.

While working in Bransholme, I got an offer to do some work in Doha Qatar. I was offered a job there back when I was in India. I returned the documents and air ticket and declined the offer. I still kept the contacts. I took an extended annual leave and went over. I landed at Doha by about 5 PM. On opening the door of the aircraft, I thought I was being put in an oven, the temperature was 43 degrees Celsius.

I was put up in a villa near the hospital. The dinner was sumptuous. The caretaker Mathew was very friendly and helpful. I told him that I would like a coffee at 6 AM and the newspaper, *Gulf News,* which is published there. I had a deep sleep and woke up by 5.30 in the morning. Thinking that the newspaper might have arrived, I came down and opened the front door. To my surprise, the front door was not locked at all. In a state of panic, I rang Mathew. He came immediately and thinking that I got the time mixed up, he said, "Sir, you said 6 o'clock for the coffee." I replied, "Yes, but why didn't you lock the door?. My passport and valuables were left on my table." After trying to conceal a wry smile he said, "Sir, we don't lock the door for almost 10 months of the year; there are only two months when we lock it - when there is sandy stormy wind from the desert." I was in Bransholme the previous day; I just envisaged the scenario if somebody went to bed without locking the door there. What a stark contrast! Later on, I noticed many cars with expensive cameras, watches etc lying on the seats. Nobody dares to touch; even for looking at them, one could end up in trouble. Law and order was instantaneous and punishment meted out swiftly without any wastage of time.

The meals were heavy and in two weeks, I put on half a stone. I realised that I had to put the brake on my feeding habits. I started cutting down on the rich food. The work was busy with a monotonous regularity of cases. After work, I went straight back to the villa since there were not many social activities. Although the authorities wanted me to stay longer, I left after six weeks.

The flight to Manchester was fully packed. I found that I was sitting next to an elderly female version of Magnus Magnusson. When she found out that she had a doctor sitting next to her, she began to conduct her own medical *Mastermind* by asking me all sorts of questions related to the various conditions she had. To escape her challenge of my medical knowledge, I politely pointed out that I was very tired and needed some sleep. In the resulting silence, aided by excellent food and alcohol, I fell from post-prandial dip into a state of narcosis.

This was shattered when I found myself being shaken awake by my travelling companion. I thought something was strange. What made me sit bolt upright was a loud commotion behind me towards the rear of the plane. I tried to concentrate on what my fellow passenger was trying to tell me. She said somebody is injured and she thought that maybe it was a hijack. In one breath, I said all my prayers and summoned up the courage to look behind me. There was a pandemonium near the rear toilets and cabin crew were scrambling around. Calling on all my reserves of courage, I went to the scene. I tried to look calm but my stomach was performing cartwheels.

However, it was not a bunch of gun-trotting extremists demanding the release of their brothers in arms, but the consternation turned out to be a ten year-old boy with a nasty gash which was bleeding profusely. He tripped in the toilet and banged his head. It was my time to take charge. I sat down holding him, applied steady pressure and used a steristrip and compression bandage. The job was done. Cabin crew did the mopping up. I returned to my seat. Shortly afterwards, the first officer came on the tannoy and thanked me. My companion was hilarious. She forced me to stand up alongside her and wave to the crowd. I felt like a puppet being manipulated by a master.

After two years in General Practice, I wrote this poem:

Metamorphosis

Went on the hospital practice,

Full of dreams and whispers;

At beck and call of men in grey suits,

Nurses and porters;

Worked like donkey days and nights,

For paltry returns.

Aspiration to perspiration and dreams to nightmare,

Cyclical changes went bizarre.

Despondent, disillusioned and made the exit.

Metamorphosis into General Practitioner smelt
fragrant.

Soon grasped FP10, FM3-symbols of GP icon.

Felt like Armstrong stepping on moon.

Alas, came the 1990 contract - Damocles sword,

Hanging on the hood of GP overworked.

Sleepless nights and unending patient demands,

Galaxy of complaints chasing all around.

24 hour care followed like shadow in slumber daze,

The *Healthcall* rang for extra help even on lazy days of grace.

When the going got worse from firm to hard,

There appeared the demon from high command;

The unplanned progeny from oblivion – *patients' charter,*

To make the GP sweat, harass and labour,

To give the community Health Council freedom to put GP in terror.

There appeared shining star on the firmament,

The nightingale -Virginia with £9 a visit,

'Take it or be damned', or else… with a threat.

Soon will there be exodus from General Practice,

Hoping to find some well-earned solace.

Prescribing

*'The young physician starts with 20 drugs for each disease, and
the old physician ends life with one drug for 20 diseases.'*

Sir William Osler

One of the important roles of any GP is medicine
management; medications – prescription, review and
monitoring. Overzealous prescribing has been going
on for centuries. Louis XIII underwent 212 enemas,
215 purgations and 47 bleedings in a single year. A
canon of the Diocese of Troyes in France was given
2190 enemas over a two year period.

The pharmaceutical industry is a global powerhouse. In
1975, while addressing the World Health Assembly,
Dr Halfdan Mahler, the WHO Director General
commented, 'Drugs not authorized for sale in the
country of origin or withdrawn from the market for
reasons of lack of safety or lack of efficacy, are
sometimes exported and marketed in developing
countries. Other drugs are promoted and advertised in
those countries for indications that are not approved
by the regulatory agencies of the countries of origin.
Products not meeting the quality requirements of the
exporting country, including products beyond their
expiry date, may be exported to developing countries
that are not in a position to carry out quality control
measures.'

The late Sir Clifford Allbutt commented, 'Poor creatures, arrant or sinful, God help them, I cannot; yet pill or potion be a comfort to them, or a hope, by all means let them have it.'

In the NHS, medical care, apart from prescription charge (which is also exempt for many) is free at the point of consumption. The consumer (the patient) is unaware of the cost involved. The water company advertisement says, 'You pay for every drop you use'. When people use gas, electricity and water, they are aware of the bills to come and use the utilities judiciously. Since the NHS is free, the service is overused, misused and abused by many.

When telephoning the doctor for a home visit, many do not think of the ramifications of the call - the doctor's time, transport and other hidden costs. The demands on the health service are unlimited while the resources are finite. The vast majority of patients who are beneficiaries of the NHS are unaware of the inadequacies of the supply. They think NHS is a bottomless pit.

For the public, the GP is the first line of defence against illness. He is the bridge between patients and the hospitals. Although patients are referred for investigations and treatment to hospitals, the GP still remains in overall charge in the long run. When acting as interpreter after receiving specialist care, the GP has a unique role in driving home important messages. Hence, the family doctor can implant knowledge about supply and demand inadequacies in the practice population to enable them to understand the intricacies of health economics.

Patients have a civic responsibility for prudent and judicious use of the usage of NHS. The government ought to improve the health education regarding the finiteness of resources. There is no point in painting a misleading picture that the overstretched, never-ending and ever-changing health demands of the nation will be met at all costs. The health of the nation depends on the wealth of the nation.

Antibiotic prescribing has always been a contentious issue for patients, the GPs and the NHS. In the good old days, doctors only issued a limited amount of medications - Aspirin for fever, mercury for syphilis and quinine for malaria and so on. The main role of the doctors was to share the burden of illness with the patient and family and to reassure them that somebody with specialist knowledge was looking after them. But it was not until 1928 that Penicillin, the first true antibiotic, was discovered by Alexander Fleming, Professor of Bacteriology at St. Mary's Hospital in London.

The public concepts have changed with the modernisation of society. Broadly, the patients have an awesome obsession for curative medicine and believe doctors should be able to produce 'a pill for every ill'. The doctor is coerced into acting as a technician. He is instrumental in prescribing hundreds of drugs, the ultimate co-benefactor is the pharmaceutical industry. In 1998, when the House of Lords released the report on antibiotic prescribing, Lord Soulsby remarked, 'Anything from 20 to 50 percent of the antibiotics prescribed are possibly unnecessary'. Although the medical profession has been trying the problem is still a challenging situation.

*　　　　　　　*　　　　　　　*

Bicycles need number-plates

The Daily *Mail*, January 15, 2008 reported that a cyclist hurling through and jumping a red traffic light, outside the House of Lords, tried to snatch the handbag of an 84 year-old lady, Tory peer Baroness Sharples. She, inspired like Lady Thatcher, delivered a sharp punch and the man fled. I wrote to Baroness Sharples and sent the article I had written and reinforced legislation to put number plates on bicycles.

During the last quarter of century, I have made some salient observations regarding bicycle riders. The majority of cyclists who use them as a conduit to get to work appear to be responsible on the road. But, significant numbers appear to be in a world of their own, paying scant respect for other road users.

Incidences observed are as follows, reminding me of the acts of the seven stages of man described by Shakespeare.

- **At first the infant mewling and puking.** It is in the hind-basket of mother. This is mom's daily trip to get bread and milk. Apart from whistling screams, fleeting cries and wetting the nappies synchronising bumpy rides, they are harmless.

- **And then the whining shining schoolboy, unwilling to school.** They ride helter-skelter, scatter the pigeons and even propel in the opposite direction in one-way streets.

- **And then the lover, sighing like a furnace, with a woeful ballad, made to mistress' eyebrow.** These are deadly, since they travel like a guided missile in phantom land and are likely to turn abruptly in any direction. They will be holding mobile phones and get into deep and heart-felt conversation, a cigarette on the lips, not concentrating on the road and holding the handle with half a finger or so.

- **Then a soldier, full of strange oaths, jealous in honour, sudden and quick in quarrel.** They just pose at red light, have a quick look and make a sudden leap, believe that the entire road is their own. These display half a cigar as a showpiece. Beware of road rage in this category. They are the likely ones to go peddling after having a few beers, again putting everybody around in mortal danger.

- **And then the justice, in fair round belly with good capon lined.** They are very tolerant, but they tend to have tunnel vision, with no hand signals at all.

- ***The sixth stage slips into the lean and slipper'd pantaloons, with spectacles on nose and pouch on side.*** These are the gentlemen on two wheels, observing all traffic rules and gesturing signals appropriately but seldom wear any protective helmets, because they can't afford to buy it with their pension, which they spend on single malt whisky.

- ***Last scene of all, is second childishness, and mere oblivion, sans teeth, sans eyes, sans everything.*** These are nocturnal creatures, bothering not to have any lights, bell or even brakes.

These show a pattern of pathetic exhibition of lamentable violation of traffic regulations and disrespect to fellow road users. Most often, the cyclists who ride erratically and cause motor vehicle accidents escape unscathed and flee scot-free. This behaviour is based on the assumption that they are not accountable, identifiable or traceable. Many are intoxicated with booze, drugs or passion.

The way forward is to make it mandatory for all cycles to be licenced, insured and taxed to bear number plates. This would make them accountable and improve the civic sense in using roads. In case of accidents, they will be treated like a motorist. Also, it would bring a broad smile to the chancellor's face.

It is the innate fear of accountability that prompts man to behave in a civilised manner.

On 9th October 2014, *The Times* reported that Sussex Crime and Police Commissioner Katy Bourne called for number plating for cyclists.

Fear lent wings to his feet.

Virgil (Roman Poet)

Public opinion

The publication **PULSE** (August 2018) reported about the plight of a surgery, where all GPs were female. There were various patient complaints about this. The Care Quality Commission also criticised the Practice. They had tried their best to recruit a male GP with no success. But the public think that the surgery is at fault.

Newspapers are keen to print public opinion about various medical issues and controversies. The internet revolt ion has transformed the public understanding of diseases and ailments. Although in theory, it is beneficial to some extent, it has its drawbacks. Ex Surgeon-Gynaecologist to the Queen, Sir John Peel, wrote in *The Times,* 'In our modern society we have an obsession that public debate will solve every problem whereas in fact it not infrequently means that the judgement of the ignorant and ill-informed takes precedence over that of those with experience and special knowledge. The practice of medicine is about caring for patients individually and their families. I have a strong feeling that too much public debate only makes matters more confused, where difficult and delicate decisions have to be made which primarily concern the individual.'

The night I slept among three ladies...

It was about seven in the evening, when I visited Edith, a pleasant, buoyant and precocious eighty-three year-old lady who had developed cellulitis of leg. Seeing me through the window, albeit the pain and discomfort, she hobbled to open the door for me. While I was writing the prescription, the heat of her prying eyes made me feel curious. Clearing her throat as a preface, she remarked, "Doctor, you don't look well, what is the matter? I think you need to see a doctor." I replied in a vague subdued muffle, "Well, I had a cough the last few days; I am not feeling that clever." Feeling shrunken and brittle, I left her house. Driving home, her voice kept ringing in my ears. I contacted my GP who arranged admission to hospital with suspected pneumonia.

Since there was no bed available, I had to wait for the call from hospital before I could set off. Finally, I landed in hospital about eleven at night. The porter took me in a wheelchair from the porch and during the sojourn to the ward, I felt like a vulnerable being making a lonely journey. When I reached the ward, there was an aura of mystic silence. The lights were dimmed and I was ushered into bed 2 in the cubicle. A nurse dropped in, checked my vital signs and left saying that the doctor will come later to see me. The curtains were drawn; feeling exhausted I collapsed into bed. The clock chimed ceremoniously twelve times breaking the uneasy silence. Feeling like a caged animal, soon I slipped into semi-narcosis.

The sleep was broken by the doctor in the form of a young petite lady with South American roots at about half past two. I consoled - better late than never. After duly examining me, she mounted a series of futile missions to extract some blood from me. The more she tried, the less enjoyable it was for me. Eventually, with some assistance from the nurse, when the mission was accomplished my elbows had turned into pink cushions. The lingering thick aroma of some oriental perfume triggered the pace of blood circulating through my temples violently, causing a thumping headache. Battered and bruised, sleep came to my rescue shortly.

The chirping of birds and some chit-chat in a hushed voice woke me up; it was quarter to seven in the morning. The smell of burnt toast wafted through my olfactory system. With eagerness I partially opened the curtain and lay feigning sleep. In a few minutes, I noticed a lady in her late sixties in a dull white nightie approaching me. She appeared fragile, remote with a pallid face and tranquil smile. Imbued in grace, she put a cup of tea beside me on the bedside cabinet. Before I could thank her, she turned around in a smooth choreographed motion. No words could be exchanged.

My brain started functioning. Who is this lady? I didn't have to think much. I could overhear the whispering conversation of ladies in my close neighbourhood, saying that a local GP was admitted last night among them. My poor plight was being debated at length by those 'expert patients'. The curiosity turned into an intricate nonplus crux that I had been admitted into a ladies' ward. What about my privacy, dignity and confidentiality?

Since 1997, government set various deadlines to end the practice of mixed wards. I wonder if Aneurin Bevan had envisaged this while founding the NHS.

*   *   *

HM Prison

Our practice used to cover HM Prison, Hull, on a regular basis. Although challenging, the job was a different facet of general practice. On Easter Monday 1994, after doing the morning rounds, I was about to leave. Suddenly an order was sent across all corridors - no movement. That went on for hours. One of the most dangerous and violent criminals, Charles Bronson, had taken the deputy governor Adrian

Wallace as hostage. The ensuing tense ordeal went on for nearly six hours. So I, along with all others, were held in captivity within our rooms. I decided to quit prison work after that.

*   *   *

In 1996, I attended a six-day course leading to a Certificate in Medical Law at the University of Glasgow. Glasgow is a port city on the River Clyde in Scotland's western Lowlands. It's famed for its Victorian and art nouveau architecture, a rich legacy of the city's 18th–20th-century prosperity due to trade and shipbuilding. Today it's a national cultural hub, home to institutions including the Scottish Opera, Scottish Ballet and National Theatre of Scotland, as well as acclaimed museums and a thriving music scene. The University of Glasgow is a public research university. Founded by papal bull in 1451, it is the fourth oldest university in the English-speaking world and one of Scotland's four ancient universities.

GPs are much more vulnerable than the hospital colleagues as far as litigation is concerned sine 95 % of patient contact is with GPs. Also the hospital set up is much more insulated while GPs come across lots on unexpected scenarios involving a multitude of people and they are responsible for the primary care team. As new laws continue to emerge and the existing ones are re-interpreted, it was of paramount importance to be well versed with medical law and its implications. The studies took part in the Gothic building of the university. I stayed at the nearby Grosvenor Hotel.

Ignorentia jursi nemo excusat which means ignorance of the law is no excuse.

The medical practice is much more complex than a simple doctor-patient relationship. The wellbeing of each and every one in society is the responsibility of everybody and the State. The state has a basic duty, based on social contract and human rights legislation to protect all citizens from harm – real or envisaged. The concepts of medical ethics have changed over the years. Health promotion and health protection have been at the forefront with overriding emphasis especially over last 50 years. The relation is triangular between doctor, patient and the state.

Every other day, the newspapers carry reports law suits, some very perplexing. The course was very thorough, methodical and updating the knowledge in medical law and ethics.

As Mason & McCall Smith put it, 'Intervention by law is too blunt a way of tackling the delicate and ethical dilemmas, which doctors have to face. Guided by personal experience and by prevailing public and professional standards, the individual must confront and resolve the day-to-day issues.'

After this course, I went on to take a Diploma in Medical Law & Ethics from the University of Glasgow.

$*$ $*$ $*$

Funny Old World

> *Always laugh when you can- it's cheap medicine.*
>
> *George Byron*

Life is full of fun, without it we would not survive.

The Independent newspaper published an article on 13 May 1997 '**Bedside manner fails to impress doctors on call**':

One 82-year-old woman called up Dr Thomas Abraham of Hull at dawn one morning complaining she had been awake since 4.30am seized with "an irresistible desire for sex". Wisely refusing to leave the security of his own bed, Dr Abraham offered her advice over the phone. He declined to visit "for reasons of personal safety."

Dr Timothy Woodman, from Gillingham, Kent, was called by a woman at 3 AM who wanted him to remove her sleeping daughter's contact lenses. He, too, declined to leave his bed.

A Birmingham GP told of being called on a Sunday evening for help with a crossword on the grounds that the answer was "a medical word", and another in Grays

Thurrock, Essex, declined to visit a patient complaining of "excess wind".

The survey, by the medical magazine *Pulse*, also records the case of a woman who walked from her home in Hornchurch, Essex, to her GP's surgery - only to ask for a home visit as her phone was broken. A British Medical Association spokeswoman said out-of-hours calls to GPs had risen fivefold over the past 20 years.

In August 2018, a consultant urologist wrote to me, 'This 19 year-old man came in as emergency after trying to perform home circumcision with a device he bought on the internet. Unfortunately, the clamp got stuck on his penis. We had to remove it under general anaesthetic'.

One day, an elderly lady with a known chronic lung problem was breathless and I did home visit. After stabilizing her, I thought I would wait a few minutes to observe and recheck her oxygen level etc. While looking out through the window into the green fields, I noticed two ivy on the windowsill. They were in special pots. On careful scrutiny, I noted the pots were Volumatics (hemispherical aids to facilitate the absorption of inhalers) which I had prescribed in the past. Human beings are innovative, imaginative and recycling all the time!

Cognac syndrome- A 23 year-old lady consulted me one evening, with a history of attending a hen night and woke up in the morning with a lump in the vagina. There were no past problems or signs of urine infection. She could not quantify amount of cognac drank (but I could still smell it). She denied any sexual encounter. This set a challenge to my medical acumen.

I asked her to do a urine sample. While waiting I scratched my brain - could be like Heineken beer 'it reaches the parts which other beers do not reach' or 'morning after the night before syndrome' or 'cognac induced vaginal oedema'??. My working diagnosis was an inflamed vaginal (Bartholin's) cyst. On examination, I recovered a glycerine suppository from her vagina. On enquiry, she was constipated for a couple of days and vaguely remembered putting it in last night without removing the cover after the drinking spree. It went in the wrong passage!

We see fake watches on the market. There were some brilliantly fake doctors. Francis Murphy was working in a meat company. One night he got an inspiration to change his vocation to be a surgeon. Of course, he had enough experience dealing with animal body parts and meat. He got some fake credentials in the name Dr AJ Murphy, whom he knew had gone abroad. He worked in Redhill Hospital as an orthopaedic registrar performing 17 operations in 4 weeks. So the medical adage came true '*A successful orthopaedic surgeon survives on brute force and bloody ignorance*'. His career ended shorty because he got into trouble operating without consent.

Even the Royals thrive on seeing the funny side of things. Prince Charles said, after unveiling a sculpture of Prince Philip, '*I now complete the process of helping my father to expose himself*'.

During a Privy Council meeting, Clare Short (then
Secretary of State for International Development) was
embarrassed that her mobile phone rang loudly. The
Queen smiled and said, *'Oh dear. I hope it wasn't anyone
important'*.

*   *   *

In 1995, I was runner-up in a national competition, for
my article on 'GP 2020 Vision', held by *DOCTOR*
publication. Primary care is as old as the human race,
from the caveman to the supersonic era. It will
continue to grow as the main vehicle of transmission
of medical care. Before 1948, medicine was practiced
mainly in a minefield of insurance schemes, voluntary
and municipal hospitals and private practice.

The World Health Organisation conference at *Alma
Atta*, USSR, in 1978 spelt out the declaration to
promote and support primary care on a global basis in
order to provide 'health for all' by 2000. The GPs' role
as explainers and interpreters of illness to patient,
family and community will gain more relevance.
Alternative medicine will continue to grow and will act
as an opiate for those disillusioned with orthodox kind.
The age of the pill will drop to fourteen. Almost all
practices will be computerised. Computers can act as
electronic GPs.

Violence against GPs will rise. Home visits will be
restricted to institutionalised patients. Litigation will be
on the increase. There will be greater restriction of

freedom of GPs. Increased number of old people will be a burden on the society. Ageism will be regarded as an offence.

*   *   *

In 1995, I had an audience with Pope John Paul II. Pope John Paul II was head of the Catholic Church and sovereign of the Vatican City State from 1978 to 2005. He was elected pope by the second papal conclave of 1978, which was called after Pope John Paul I, who died after 33 days in office. Rome, the eternal and extraordinary city is a mixture of history and legend, from a small village to the capital of boundless empire, founded by Romulus in 753 BC. As cradle of Christianity, it experienced periods of anarchy and decadence but rose up in grand splendour between 16th and 17th centuries. The Forum, located in the heart of the city, bursting with sanctuaries, halls and markets, was the grand religious, political and commercial nucleus of Rome. The **Circus Maximus** was an arena where two and four-wheeled chariots ran amok with the deafening noise of horses' galloping hooves. The **Colosseum**, the Flavian amphitheatre capable of holding 50,000 spectators, was the location where the gladiators spilt their blood in thirsty fights. The Sistine Chapel is the everlasting testament of the genius of Michelangelo. The vault contains the majestic and magnificent frescoes and paintings - among them the greatest works of art – The Creation of Adam and The Last Judgement

I received the Holy Communion from Pope John Paul II at St Peter's Basilica, the largest matrix church in the Christian world, the seat of main liturgical functions of the pope. The towering dome is 133 metres tall and 41 metres in diameter, with the interior divided by ogives and decorated with stuccoes and cartoni. It has 45 altars, 11 chapels and is laid out over 3 naves divided by sturdy pillars with niches that house a legion of statues of saints and pontiffs. The Colonnade by Gian Bernini embraces the basilica. The interior is full of masterpieces, lavishly decorated by mosaics, gold plating and precious marble features, studded with paintings and medallions.

*   *   *

In 1995, I was totally unaware of the American footballer OJ Simpson, until I was drawn into his trial which had lot of parallels with any GP's struggles after any serious allegation. I became addicted to the unfamiliar occupation of watching the televisual, long-running soap opera. What struck me was the tragic case of Dr Mathew Shiu, a GP who was charged with alleged rape after a complaint by a woman whom he examined in the surgery after he had invited the husband to stay with her. The sordid and sensational media bandwagon was too much for him. He took his own life; the forensic evidence which evolved later proved that he was innocent. A GP facing any charge is put on public display in the press and becomes the dish of the day in every pub and shop.

Michael Josephson, a legal ethicist commented, 'The OJ trial is the Chernobyl of racial justice with incredible fallout on an uneasy nation'.

'Not only did we play the race card, we played it from the bottom of the deck.'

Robert Shapiro (Simpson's Ex-Attorney)

Escalating racial rhetoric, inside and outside the courtroom, dominated the trial's final days and set the stage for a divisive verdict. Even before the verdict, it was evident how passionately the Simpson case pressed upon the sore spots of the American psyche.

1371 GPs, cleared after service committee hearings in 1994 alone, might have felt the same way. The naivety of allegations, inordinate delays, the time loss, the cost and above all the emotional trauma – all resemble the fallout after a nuclear accident like Chernobyl.

11

Rural Run

'City people make most of the fuss about the charms of country life.'

Mason Cooley

In 1995, I got appointed to take over a single-handed rural dispensing practice in the outskirts of Hull. I had about 2700 patients of which nearly 20 percent were over 75. Three surgeries were spread over 210 square miles. Most patients were very friendly and welcoming. As the news spread that I got the practice, the phone never stopped ringing; lots of people from the local Kerala community invited us for celebration parties.

Roos and Albrough surgeries were reasonable in layout and size. Burton Pidsea surgery was basically composed of two rooms, in the high street, adjacent to the post office. It reminded me of Dr Julian Hart's comments, when he worked in the mining village of Glyncorrwg, South Wales in 1961. '…two common features of industrial general practice; the seedy front parlour surgery in the GP's own home. And the squalid shop on the high street with a half-painted glass front, staffed only by a harassed GP's wife.'

Winter was harsh. Only the main roads were treated and de-iced, that too not frequent enough. Due to a lack of, or dangerous, footpaths, people tended to walk on the roads. Cars played dodgems on the roads. Gritters and snow-ploughs were rare sights. House visits were immensely difficult due to access problems in narrow country lanes. Many times, I had to depend on the generosity and benevolence of local farmers who volunteered to transform their tractors into makeshift ambulances to ferry patients into surgery or ferry me into their homes. General practice in rural areas was a different ball game compared to urban areas. In Germany and Sweden, it is compulsory to put 'winter tyres' made up of special type of rubber and different tread. Japan, Iceland and some Scandinavian countries also heat roads up. We are far behind them.

One of the most memorable people I met was Harry Jackson MBE. To me, he was a great cricketer, guide, friend and philosopher. In the year of 1931, King George V was the monarch, the Highway Code was introduced and the Empire State Building was completed. In Test Matches, Bradman scored 223 & 152 against West Indies and 112 against South Africa. In June that year, in the remote village of Burton Agnes (East Yorks) Harry Jackson was borne.

Harry started as a player aged 15 when Humbleton Cricket Club was formed in 1946. He had various fielding positions - player, umpire, secretary, treasurer and groundsman and still going strong as groundsman. His longevity of service to cricket of seventy years is enviable and has set a leading example for the younger generations, which is hard to beat. He is known locally as 'Mr Humbleton Cricket'.

The groundsman's role is usually unseen and seldom appreciated. The metamorphosis of turning a track into a good cricket pitch is never ending. The painful process involves getting rid of worms, add fertilisers, frequent rolling, spiking, scarifying, reseeding and cutting. While the play and players are seasonal, the groundsman works perennially. As David Gower commented, 'It's like watching a swan. What you see on the surface bears no relation to the activity going on underneath.'

Outside cricket, Harry served the in Royal Observer Corps for 32 years from 1960 in the 'cold war' era. His main role was to warn the public of the threat of nuclear attack. In 1984, he received an award for outstanding service to ROC from the Lord Lieutenant. He received Service to Sport Award from East Riding County Council in 1999 and Outstanding Service to Cricket Award from Yorkshire Cricket Board in 2010. The pinnacle of his achievement was when he was presented the **MBE** by Her Majesty the Queen in 2003 for his services to cricket and the community.

Harry attributed his success to the unfathomable support of his wife Kathleen. While players and officials usually get all the glamour and glitter, lest we forget the yeoman contributions of this legend.

Cricket is battle, service, sport and art.

Douglas Jardine

These words are true to the last syllable in Harry's case. As he is continuing to offer his service to cricket, I wish him all the luck so that he will hit a century.

I learned a lot of humanity by closely interacting with the elderly. I made arrangements with nursing homes that I would visit them on a fortnightly basis. I made a list of all the super-elderly (over 75) and made a habit of dropping in their houses once every six weeks. Often I ended up sharing a cup of tea and hot scone with them while listening to a running commentary of events since the last visits. The oldest driver in the villages was a 93 year-old gentleman. I developed a penchant to meet the over 100s and share their secret weaponry of longevity.

I was enjoying the practice well. Things were sailing smoothly. A few months later, I received a demand note from the Inland Revenue for the tax from my previous partnership, since my ex-partner had entered into a voluntary arrangement of paying off debts. At that time, partners were jointly and severally liable for the taxation purposes. It was a shock to the system, since I had duly paid my share of the tax. I was left with no other choice but to agree with the revenue to pay off the outstanding arrears on a monthly basis.

*　　　　　　　*　　　　　　　*

I recall a puzzling encounter. It was late morning; the surgery was coming to a close. The receptionist told me, "There is a lady called Jane to see you."

"Is she a medical rep?"

"No, she said it a private matter."

"OK, you can send her in please."

Jane was in her mid-twenties with a pale complexion, shoulder-length auburn hair and beaming smile. Leaning forward, she said, "You know Mrs Jones who died last month? She was my aunt."

"I am sorry; my heartfelt condolences."

"She celebrated her 87th birthday a month before her death. She died peacefully in her sleep. We gave her a quiet family funeral that is what she wanted." She said it all in one breath like a rehearsed speech.

I listened patiently with deep concentration. "Is there anything I can do for you?"

'Well, I don't know how to put it...' She made a vain attempt to mask her emotions but the spreading pallor on her face told the story. "Please feel free. I am here to help."

'Doctor, she always used to talk about you. She thought very highly about you. The thing is...we were going through her belongings and I saw your name."

A suffocating stillness permeated in the room. She went on. "She left something for you and a few others. But the family feels that she did not consult anybody."

Suddenly I felt vulnerable and weak. My mind was travelling like a spaceship encircling the globe. I was being drawn into a moral and ethical dilemma. Was it right to accept or not? The million-dollar question was - what was the mystery gift? Should I ring my medical defence society?

A gusty wind rattled the windows distracting my attention. Outside, dark clouds gathered momentum and were fiercely competing with each other. A fear of the unknown gripped me like a chill.

I regained my composure and replied. "The best thing is for me to give you the details of my solicitor. If your family solicitor can contact him. That is the most appropriate action."

'Doctor, do you know what it is?"

"I haven't got a clue. I think the best bet would be to leave it to solicitors."

The telephone rang. I put it on hold and said goodbye to her. I rang my solicitor and explained. He said he would deal with it.

Three weeks later, a cardboard box arrived in the surgery. There was a thank you card inside saying, 'Thank you for all what you have done for me. Regards. Mrs Jones.'

Although eager, with self-imposed calmness I opened the box. Inside it was a china pot, predominantly white with a map of the world painted in deep blue. The lid was missing. Turning it around, I noticed an oblong crack, which nearly bisected the world map, symbolising breaking the boulevard of my imagination and dreams.

I did a test; filled it with hot water. This confirmed my initial diagnosis that this was a topless, leaking tea pot. For health and safety reasons, it went straight into the bin. In short, the gap between the cup and the lip remained the same.

*   *   *

I was one of the two GPs who did vasectomies requested by other GPs in the area. Because it was done under local anaesthetic, I used to be vocal as well to distract the patient during the operation. It was a theatrical and gladiatorial performance at times.

One day, after performing a vasectomy on a 35 year-old man, I commented, "'No jot of blood' has spilled."

He asked me what that was about. I told him that it is from Shakespeare's play - *The Merchant of Venice*. He had no idea. I narrated the story. Merchant Antonio borrowed money from Shylock. Shylock demanded a pound of flesh as security if he could not repay the money on time. Unfortunately, Antonio could not repay on time and begged for clemency. Shylock, being brutal, took him to court demanding the 'pound of flesh'. The counsel for Antonio, Portia made the exuberant speech in the court. 'This bond doth give thee here no jot of blood; the words expressly are 'a pound of flesh'. Since it was impossible to execute, Shylock had to give up. This was a figurative way of referring to a harsh demand or spiteful penalty. It was an epitome of sensational bargain with a hint of archetypal vengeance. My reading of Shakespeare as a school boy, paid off.

*   *   *

In 1996, I attended the International College of Surgeons 3-day conference at Kanyakumari, a coastal town in the state of Tamil Nadu on India's southern tip. Jutting into the Laccadive Sea, the town was known as Cape Comorin during British rule and was popular for pilgrimage sites - Bagavathi Amman Temple, dedicated to a consort of Shiva and Our Lady of Ransom Church, a centre of Catholicism. It is the point of blending of three seas - Bay of Bengal, Indian Ocean and Arabian Sea. It is the only place in the country where we can enjoy the natural phenomena of sunrise and sunset happening in the Sea.

The scene was very clear and mind blowing. It looked like sun coming from the sea. The point of three seas meeting together is known as 'Triveni Sangamam'. In the full-moon day in the month of chithirai (Tamil month) the sunset and the moon rise at the opposite side and can be seen, an awesome natural phenomenon. The multi-coloured sand is a unique feature of the beach here. Kanyakumari was once referred to as the Alexandria of the East.

*   *   *

Did Not Attend Syndrome

One of the ongoing problems is patients not turning up to keep appointments.

As per NHS England's January 2019 figures, more than 15 million general practice appointments are being wasted each year because patients do not turn up and fail to warn surgeries that they will not be attending.

There are around 307 million sessions scheduled with GPs, nurses, therapists and other practice staff every year and 5% – one in 20 – are missed without enough notice to invite other patients. That works out as around 15.4 million missed slots.

Of these, around 7.2 million are with busy family doctors, which adds up to more than 1.2 million GP hours wasted each year – the equivalent of over 600 GPs working full-time for a year.

Each appointment costs an average of £30, putting the total cost to the NHS at more than £216 million on top of the disruption for staff and fellow patients, that could pay for the annual salary of 2,325 full time GPs, 224,640 cataract operations, 58,320 hip replacement operations, 216,000 drug treatment courses for Alzheimer's, the annual salary of 8,424 full-time community nurses. On the other hand, if a GP does not turn up at surgery, the complaints machinery will be working overtime and the men in grey suits will spring into action post-haste. The waiting lists are getting longer partly because of these 'phantom patients' who do not keep appointments. In this era, where each household has three or more phones, there is no justification whatsoever not to inform the GP or hospital well ahead of time if somebody cannot keep the appointment. The Doctor-Patient Partnership launched a 'Keep it or Cancel it' campaign without much success.

Dentists and vets charge a fee if somebody does not keep their appointment. We need a system of accountability from the public. If the NHS is for the people, it ought to be by the people and of the people.

*　　　　　　　*　　　　　　　*

Teaching

'I desire no other epitaph... than the statement that I taught medical students, as I regard this as by far the most useful and important work I have been called upon to do.'

Sir William Osler, Canadian Physician

Teaching is a vocation which was close to my heart all my life. I had various roles with Leeds Medical School - Tutor, Honorary Lecturer and MB ChB examiner. I used to teach fourth year students placed at surgery for two weeks at a time. Each of them stayed with me at my home and spent all their time with me at surgery, home visits and meetings. In the leading article of the *British Medical Journal* dated 20 December 1952, Hugh Clegg remarked about GPs, 'Unless something is done to re-orient graduate and undergraduate training to medicine as it is today - more exact and exacting, more of an applied science than an empirical art, the GP risks becoming what Gerald Horner called a mere medical shop-walker.'

The roles and responsibilities of the teaching were complex, time-consuming and challenging at times. I had to prepare a provisional timetable of activities for students before their arrival, allowing sufficient flexibility for variation taking into consideration the particular needs of the students. On arrival, I had to discuss with them learning objectives of the attachment and any personal objectives the students wanted. This had to be re-assessed in the middle and at the end of each attachment to ensure the objectives have been achieved. I had to observe students interacting with patients and give them feedback on their performance. Some patients were very much willing to be interviewed by the students, making my life easier. In teaching consultation skills, three methods were routinely used - student observing tutor, tutor observing student and solo consultation by the student. A subsequent appraisal followed. I used to update teaching skills by attending training seminars and courses periodically. Overall, it was thoroughly enjoyable and rewarding with great job satisfaction.

*　　　　　　　*　　　　　　　*

Andropause

Hundreds of middle-aged women see their GPs attributing their problem to the climacteric and seek help. Universally, women get sympathy at home, work and in society for menopausal miseries. In reality, a fair number of men of similar age group consult GPs due to ailments coming under similar umbrella of symptoms.

The Oxford Dictionary defines climacteric as (a) a period of life when fertility and sexual activity are on the decline (b) a critical period of life (c) a crisis period. In ancient Greek literature, a grand climacteric has been identified in men at age 63. There have been different views regarding the age of onset ranging from 38, 57 and 63. Havelock Ellis' description is worth noting, 'In many cases, such a period occurs even near the age of 38. The man suddenly realises that the period of expandery powers has reached its limits, even that there is a comparative failure of powers, this also manifesting itself in the sexual sphere, and by sudden revulsion of feeling that he may begin to feel that he is no longer a young but an old man.'

In women, the climacteric coincides with the shutting down of the procreative factory since nature does not want her to carry on that big burden, when her physical faculties are on the decline. But man is capable of carrying on regardless, procreating even into his eighties or nineties. It is worth noting Goethe fell in love with a young girl at the age of 74. Most recently, as CNN reported on 3rd April 2020, Formula 1 mogul, Bernie Ecclestone, was on track to become a father again at the tender age of 89. He quipped, "I don't see there is any difference between being 89 and 29. You have got the same problems."

The signs are less typical and demarcated but the symptoms are similar. The symptoms are gain in weight, hot flushes, sweating, palpitations, lethargy, irritability, mood disturbances, impaired concentration, depression, prostatic symptoms and sleep disturbances. Psycho-sexual symptoms include diminished libido and impotence. Sexual aberrations like predisposition to young girls and exhibitionism ('park offences') have been described. In most cases, testosterone (the male hormone) is low, which can be treated.

*　　　　　*　　　　　*

In 1996, I went to India to celebrate my father's 75th birthday. I kept it as total surprise to him. All the planning was done meticulously by consulting my mum and brothers. In the morning, my father was having his daily walk at about 8.30. I went up to him and said, "A friend of mine has invited all of us this afternoon; can you get ready and dressed by 10.30?" I heard him asking my mum the details. Mum said she did not know any details and that I also had told her to stay ready. By 10.15 a people carrier van arrived, whose driver was Joe, son of my school-mate. We set off and picked up my brother and family on the way.

The winding twisty roads are paved but narrow, with some curvy and steep parts. Starting from Kochi, the drive is 72 miles long. One can experience a beautiful cool drive through a natural forest, with many refreshing waterfalls. The road was certainly breath-taking and it has a fearsome reputation. The road is blind in some places and there are a lot of trucks and buses that seem to drive as if they own the road. Adimali was 20 miles to Munnar and the last place you can spot a decent restaurant on the way. The final 20 miles took about an hour. Around 15 miles from Adimali, we started seeing the tea plantations on both sides of the road and a panoramic view of the Western Ghats. The view is extremely beautiful during the early mornings. While driving on the road, you are ensnared in the sweet fragrance of the fresh tea leaves from innumerable tea plantations. But the road to Munnar is narrow with lots of bends and curves. The road is potentially dangerous, especially for who are not familiar with the topography. At times, the road becomes covered in fog, which makes it impossible to see even with your fog lamps on. There have been lots of fatal accidents on this terrain.

Munnar is a town in the Western Ghats mountain range in Kerala state. A hill station and former resort for the British Raj elite, it is surrounded by rolling hills dotted with tea plantations established in the late 19th century. Eravikulam National Park is the home of the endangered mountain goat Nilgiri Tahr. There was Lakkam Waterfalls, hiking trails and 2,695m-tall Anamudi Peak.

The barbeque started with a 'mountain cocktail' befitting the mountainous area we were in. It composed of Vermouth, lemon juice, white of egg and Canadian Club Whisky. Plenty of snacks - banana chips, cashew nuts, Bombay mixture and pappad were at our disposal. The main dishes were veal escalope, grilled chicken with peanut sauce and lobster mayonnaise supported with stuffed cabbage leaves, carrots, Pilav rice and chappathi. Carrot halva and rice pudding concluded the treat.

On the way back, we visited Thekkady, the whole area was under his jurisdiction in his heydays. The motel was very nice. The restaurant manager, John, hailed from a village 5 miles from my home with many common relatives and friends. So, he was very keen to establish a warm rapport.

John set out a special corner for us to relax. He asked me what my favourite drink was. Both myself and my dad preferred whisky. He said he get us the drink 'Whisky Toddy'. Toddy is the local name for palm wine. I thought it did not mix well; anyway we waited. He brought the drink and said with grin, "This will warm you up nicely." The drink was not exactly what I expected. It was whisky, one teaspoon sugar, hot water and served with a slice of lemon. The drink reached all parts of the body in a haste producing a state of flushing and warm feeling, which was in desperate need in the cold climate (the outside temperature was 2 degrees Celsius that night).

Later on, John gave me a masterclass on making cocktails. He had a degree in culinary science and had worked at a five-star hotel in Calcutta in the past. He gave a running commentary of all the feats and achievements of his career. A cocktail mixer pretends to be a magician who compounds his recipes according to a secret formulae producing delicious delightful drinks to the utmost discriminating palates. He showed the tools of his trade like a whining schoolboy proudly exhibiting his toys to his mates. The cocktail cabinet was made of mahogany. Equipment composed of a shaker (two nickel containers fitting into each other), mixing glass (large tumbler), mixing spoon (long-handled tea spoon), strainer, lemon squeezer, muddler (implement for crushing) and measure (to measure volume). We went to bed by 11 at night. At the breakfast table, my mum appeared a bit sulky. When I enquired to my wife Mary told me she lost the watch overnight. I had bought a watch at Manchester airport and gifted her the previous week when I arrived in India. I did not want that to spoil the occasion. I just told my mum, "Don't worry; I will get another watch on the way home." I told John what happened. He said the staff are wonderful and trustworthy and to leave the matter with him. A couple of hours later, John came back with the watch. The culprit was a monkey who was a regular thief and hoarded things at his night shelter. He would have got in through the bathroom window which was left open. Mum had left it there while having a shower. Overall, the trip was thoroughly enjoyable, tracing back nostalgic memories of the days gone past.

*   *   *

In 1997, I went to Arles, Southern France, to meet the oldest person on earth, Madame Jeanne Calment. She was 122 years-old, born in 1875. Vincent Van Gogh was her neighbour. She had an uneventful childhood. At age 21, she got married to her second cousin who had a drapery industry locally. Her only daughter died aged 36 due to pleurisy. According to her narration, during World War II, German soldiers slept in her room but 'did not take anything away'. Her husband died at 73.

In 1965, aged 90 she signed a 'Life Estate Agreement' with local notary public Andre-Francois Raffray, selling her house to him in exchange of right of occupancy and monthly 2500 Francs (£380) until her death. The notary died in 1995 having paid a lot of money. She did 'Carry On Living'.

She outlived 21 French Presidents. She had been cycling around Arles till the age of 90. On meeting her, the first thing she commented in French was, "You have come a long way." She appeared to be in good spirits. Although she was visually impaired due to cataracts, when I gave her a bottle of Port, her eyes lit up. She used to drink nearly a quarter bottle of port a day and smoke 20 cigarettes daily till the age of 117 when she stopped smoking. She said she got bored and re-started smoking on her 118th birthday. When she got into *The Guinness Book of Records* as the oldest living person on earth at 120 years and 238 days, her doctor Victor Lebre commented, "Now she has a few goals to fulfil." She was the modern day Methuselah. What an enigma of God's creation! I still carry in my doctor's bag my picture of her. When some elderly patients talk despondently about their problems and feel like giving up, I tell them, "You are still a spring chicken' and give them shock therapy by showing the photograph. This has really worked to cheer them up and boost their morale.

The better living and working conditions over the last few decades have improved the longevity of life. The elderly are more vulnerable to various ailments. They need society's support to keep them active and well. They should not be penalised or patronized because of their age. One key problem is loneliness. Many old people live on their own. Many who live with their partners, have deviated in their paths and outlook of life and still feel isolated and live parallel lives under the same roof. Health and happiness are intimately related as hands in gloves.

*   *   *

It was reported that on New Year's Day 1997, the body of a 61 year-old lady was brought into a hospital mortuary. She had been pronounced dead by the GP. The mortuary attendant noticed that she was breathing and called the crash team who took over the management and the lady recovered in the hospital. This was a lesson for all of us. Often GPs are called at unearthly hours of the night to certify somebody's death. The usual spectacle is relatives crowding around the body in a shocked state, perplexed regarding the death and speculating the corollary of events to follow, especially when the death is unexpected. The GP has to do a clinical examination and make on the spot decision. The incident was thought-provoking, challenging and a learning opportunity.

Pliny the Elder wrote in *Historia Naturalis* in first century AD 'So uncertain is men's judgement that they cannot determine even death itself'.

*   *   *

We moved to Hessle in 1997, close to Humber Bridge. This was the longest suspension bridge in the world till 1998 opened by Her Majesty Queen Elizabeth II on 24 June 1981. It is 1.4 miles long and 1.5 million vehicles pass through per year. It was designed by Sir Ralph Harrison who is the son of Sir Ralph Harrison, who designed Sydney Harbour Bridge. Now, Akashi Kaikyo Bridge in Japan is the longest suspension bridge in the world. The week of moving was one when the world stood still marked by the death of Princess Dianna.

The typical working day started with a cup of tea and quick shower, dropping children to school and driving to surgery. Morning surgery - 30 patients, then 2 hours administration- dealing with prescriptions, hospital letters, referrals, health authority matters, patient related matters, financial issues, staff problems and sickness. Then home visits usually 4 to 6 per day. Because of the rural spread of patients, lots of time was lost in travel. Evening surgery was 25 patients. On finishing surgery, the smiling secretary handed over a 'take away'- a carrier bag full of insurance and social security forms etc. In spite of all the heavy workload, I won the Health Authority Incentive Scheme payment of £3000 for judicious and prudent prescribing during 1996-97, which was ploughed back into the development of the practice.

In 1997, an overworked GP who become addicted to amphetamines was sentenced by Magistrate Charles Ley. 'You are a man who put a lot into your profession as a doctor and into public life. In fact you are a classic example of a man who has strived to do so much. In doing so, have pressed your own self-destruct button.' He was fined £1200 and reported to the General Medical Council. This struck me – I did not want to end up like that.

In trying to fulfil the profession's and public's expectations, I tried to squeeze too much into my work schedule. I carried an unbelievable burden of frustrating responsibilities. Loss of time in travelling between surgeries and callouts took a heavy toll on me. I was struggling to beat the clock day in and day out. Financial worries were looming and threatening to engulf me. Roman poet Virgil wrote 2000 years back, *'Non omnia possumus omnes'* (We can't do everything). I resigned from the practice.

12

The Pariah

'Victory has a thousand fathers but defeat is an orphan.'

John F Kennedy

Most from the Kerala community in Hull treated me
and my family as social pariah, ostracized completely
like a leper. The very same people, who kept on
inviting us for parties when I got the rural practice in
1997, were the leaders in treating me like anathema.
We were not informed of any social functions; nobody
invited us to parties or any celebrations. The only
persons who stood by me throughout were the late Dr
Joseph Austin, who was GP at Bilton and Dr John
Zachariah from Scunthorpe. In olden days when
society was far less inclusive and more orthodox, a
social pariah was somebody who was excommunicated
from society, and everybody from that society either
considered him undesirable or was forced to
disassociate with him by the village elder and decision
makers. Some would avoid eye contact and slip away at
shopping centres. Some dared not even to park near
my car, although there was an empty slot. There were

sordid sensational bandwagons of whispering campaigns targeted to discredit me from various corners. Once, a prominent showman in the church, pulled a £5 note and flashed it, looking around. and put in the collection bag which came around during the mass. He turned around to make sure everybody had seen his 'donation' and suddenly saw me sat just behind him. Instantly, he developed 'wry neck' and kept still till the end of the mass without a flicker of movement of his head and neck.

'Be careful not to practice your righteousness in front of others to be seen by them. If you do, you will have no reward from your Father in heaven. So when you give to the needy, do not announce it with trumpets, as the hypocrites do in the synagogues and on the streets, to be honoured by others.'

Matthew 6:1-4

We stopped going to church at Hessle after a while and started attending St Charles Church in Hull. I learnt that two people conducted parties to celebrate my downfall. We got nasty anonymous letters in the post, which were delivered in the porch by the postman. So, I put a letterbox outside the gate and used to collect it myself so that the rest of the family were kept out of this postal attack. My children used to get mocked at school with cryptic clues about their dad. I told my family, "Money makes the world go round. Anyway, they don't pay our mortgage or water bills; so don't bother; get on with our life." All the locals who knew me and so many of my ex-patients contacted me offering support. Some wrote in *Hull Daily Mail* supporting me from the bottom of their hearts.

'Those who dare to fail miserably can achieve greatly.'

John F Kennedy

One day, I had parked the car opposite Dr Wajahat Hussain's surgery on Anlaby Road and went to Hull Royal Infirmary Library. On return, he saw me and called me in for a chat. Hearing my plight, he commented, "We Moslems, help others in distress, it is considered a duty in our religion."

I said, "Broadly speaking Christianity and Islam are not far apart; but some people use religion as a make-up and showpiece for social climbing." He enquired whether I would be interested in joining his practice and offered me the job. Later on, I joined his practice.

*   *   *

Hospital doctors need training in general practice.

'In general practice, patients stay and diseases come and go. In hospitals, diseases stay and patients come and go.'

Heath I. BMJ 1995, 311:373

While GPs have sailed through the waters of hospital specialities and deal with all specialities on a day to day basis, general practice is unchartered territory for hospital doctors. Significant difficulties occur in patient care due to hospital doctors' poor understanding of the *modus operandi* of GPs.

Ninety-five percent of patients' contact is with GPs and most of the issues are dealt with at primary care level. Only a small percentage needs secondary care involvement like admissions or referrals. Admissions tend to cause much friction between GPs and hospital doctors. A few years back, I was doing a night visit at 2 AM. The patient was a 23 year-old lady, a single parent with a 2 year-old daughter, living on her own on the 5th floor of a tower block. Clinical picture was appendicitis. When I requested admission, the hospital doctor was rather insisting on rectal examination findings. The doctor was purely checking the possible diagnosis and not visualising the predicament of the GP who assessed the case and made the decision that the patient cannot be managed in her own home in the middle of the night and needed hospitalisation. This is due to tunnel vision of the specialist doctor and failing to visualise the danger in that procedure, which could turn out to career threatening in that situation. In my experience, there have been various other similar examples over the years.

Often, patients view the hospital as a transit lounge since they know that they are there only for a limited time and are well aware they will go back to the GP shortly. Also, many patients talk highly about their GPs. This attitude of patients can irritate many hospital doctors since they feel undervalued and underestimated for their services. For the hospital doctor, dealing with a patient lasts a few days or weeks but for a GP, the commitment is lifelong till retirement or death. If two people have to ride a horse, one has to sit in the back. Naturally, the horse prefers the familiar rider than the short-term one.

While a hospital doctor has thorough knowledge of the speciality he works in, a GP has a broad working knowledge of all conditions affecting all ages and extending over all specialities. Moreover, a GP is not just clinician but has various other roles - family practitioner, counsellor, disease interpreter, administrator, social worker, gatekeeper, primary care leader and so on. The hospital doctor's responsibility often ends with the discharge letter. Also, in the hospital setting, the burden is shared and the buck stops with the consultant. For a GP, the buck starts and stops with him.

A group from the European Working Party in Family Practice (EQuiP), involving over 20 European colleges of primary care, has found that quality of care at the interface between general practice and specialists needs much improvement. Many patients feel that they are left in limbo when care is being transferred from one branch to another. The European Task Force on Quality in General Practice (EUROPEP) has developed an instrument to measure patients' evaluation of quality in general practice. Also, benchmarking of hospitals has been in force over many years. With the rapid advent of social media, patients have become much more knowledgeable about their health care and rights. The *General Practice Forward View* set up a working group in September 2016 to (a) improve communication between primary and secondary care and (b) include new measures in the NHS Standard Contract to improve processes across the interface and (c) identify and share best practice and innovative ways of working.

One of the key recommendations by EQuiP is that specialists should be trained in the patterns of diseases, signs and symptoms within primary care system as well as those presenting to specialist practice. All trainees should have appropriate training and insight into possible organisational problems at the primary-secondary care interface from both patients' and providers' perspectives. These can only be achieved by spending enough time in general practice.

If two years hospital medicine is part of GP training, in my view, every hospital specialist doctor ought to spend at least one month per year in general practice. Rather than viewing 'my patient' and 'your patient', we all need to view it as 'our patient' and the medical profession needs to work 'hand in glove' among all branches and cadres to achieve the common goal of best possible holistic patient care.

*   *   *

1999 - I met and had a discussion Archbishop Desmond Tutu, South African anti-apartheid and human rights activist, when he came for Hull 700 celebrations. To shake hands with a Nobel Prize winner was an experience of a life-time. Rowena, my daughter, had the opportunity to give him a bouquet. He is an honorary doctor of a number of leading universities in the USA, Britain and Germany. Desmond Tutu had formulated his objective as 'a democratic and just society without racial divisions'. He set forward the following as minimum demands - equal civil rights for all, abolition of existing passport laws, a common system of education and the cessation of forced deportation from South Africa to the so-called 'homelands'.

He was honoured with the Peace Prize for his opposition to South Africa's brutal apartheid regime. He was saluted by the Nobel Committee for his clear views and his fearless stance, characteristics which had made him a unifying symbol for all African freedom fighters. Attention was once again directed at the nonviolent path to liberation. The Peace Prize award made a big difference to Tutu's international standing, and was a helpful contribution to the struggle against apartheid. The broad media coverage made him a living symbol in the struggle for liberation, someone who articulated the suffering and expectations of South Africa's oppressed masses. I had read his books before I met him. His striking quotes impressed me:

'My humanity is bound up in yours, for we can only be human together.'

'Do your little bit of good where you are, it's those little bits of good put together that overwhelm the world.'

*   *   *

Crude Compensation Culture

In 2000, the world celebrated the millennium. After working in the NHS for 15 years, I had a look at our society's way to lean towards the compensation craze. A consortium of solicitors were campaigning to encourage patients to sue GPs alleging to 'prescribe negligently' for depression. A significant percentage of public suffer from depression, the vast majority is reactive and the rest endogenous. Reactive depression is triggered by events like death in the family, physical ailments, domestic problems, financial worries etc.

Most GPs are good enough to diagnose and treat it within primary care settings. Drug therapy is only part of managing depression and GPs often assess the duration of treatment with periodic reviews.

Yet some tactics by solicitors hunting for medical negligence are lists of people with possible injuries bought from market research companies, people involved in accidents invited for meetings at hotels, leaflets and social media encouraging patients to sue.

We have a judicial system that has to be used in a civilised and controlled manner. The growing tendency to rush to courts for anything and everything is diabolical, drastic and dangerous. There are ever-increasing examples of people suing doctors for all sorts of reasons. A man diagnosed as HIV positive was told that on further testing he was negative. He sues. It is well known fact that false positive reactions occur in HIV tests. A man diagnosed as having advanced cancer, was given an estimate of life expectancy of six months. With intensive treatment, he got better, only to sue doctor two months after the deadline has passed for doing everything to prolong his life.

The ordinary patient has only one desire - to get better. He does not care much how this is achieved. Medicine is claimed to be based on science but in reality, science plays only a small part in many cases. The standard of medical conduct - both intra and inter-professional, has become more sordid and commercialised in the last half-century since the inception of the NHS.

To the conscientious and competent doctors, times and systems make little difference as far as professional service is concerned. We do our best for the patient in the given circumstances. In the discharge of duties, mistakes can happen. Those who have been wronged should be compensated; no body disputes that.

A judge remarked, "The notion of simple bad luck has just gone out of the window, but some people don't seem to understand when they have had good luck." Like fast foods, fast drug philosophy has crept into our culture; for every ill the public expects a pill. If patients do not get better, many turn to the legal system. The bottom line is the public has to understand and accept that sometimes suffering is inevitable and unavoidable.

The 16th century philosopher John Owen rightly remarked, 'God and the doctor we adore alike, but only when in danger; the danger over, both are alike requited, God is forgotten and the doctor is slighted.'

MSN News, 18 August 2009, reported that Mrs Mary Raimo, 76 year-old lady sued Tesco because a pineapple fell on her neck from the rack. The way the justice system operates can be mind-blowing at times. The *Daily Express* (12 March 2014) reported this case. Nazier Din, a 44 year-old businessman from Bury, had a brick thrown through his window by a lout causing £2500 damage. Nobody was prosecuted. He put up a sign on the boarded up window: 'A dirty pervert drug dealing grass did this'. The prime suspect went to police saying the sign 'offended' him. Although, he taped over the word pervert, police arrested him for hurting the brick-thrower's feelings. After caution, Mr Din had his DNA and fingerprints put on the national database. His legal bill of £1000 added insult to injury. Who is the real victim?

13

Annus Horribilis

'We must accept finite disappointment,

But we must never lose infinite hope.'

Martin Luther King

On Monday 7th May 2001, at five past seven in the morning, the phone rang. It was the manager from the care home saying that my daughter Teresa had not turned up for work. I said I heard her opening the garage about 6.20, so she should have been there. She kept her bike in the garage and I could always hear when the garage door opened. She was always punctual at work. So I felt something was odd. I got changed immediately and drove the route she normally takes. Soon, I came back home and alerted Mary, Thomas and Rowena. Then I walked into the Humber Bridge area called 'Little Switzerland' to check whether she could have taken a different route through the woodlands. There was nothing to find. I returned home, rang the care home again. They said she still had not turned up. My immediate thought was whether she was abducted on her way etc because she appeared fine at 9 o'clock the previous night. She had come to my room and asked, "Dad, have you got anything to type?" She used to do lot of typing for me since she was much faster. I gave her an article to type and when she was about to complete, I went up to her to make some final amendments. A few minutes later, she dropped it into my room and gave me £3, saying that she had borrowed it from my drawer couple of days back. I said, "Don't be silly; no need to return that; anyway, thanks a lot." She smiled, gave me a hug and left.

Both Mary and myself rang her on her mobile a few times; it was going to voicemail; we left so many messages to ring back etc. Then, I rang the police. The police took all the details over the phone and a policeman called at our house soon after. The Humber coastguard and the RAF helicopter from Leconfield also started searching. The police rang later in the evening to say that a bike has been found at the Humber foreshore near Dunston shipyard. A sudden spell of gloom and doom permeated on hearing that.

The police underwater search unit started searching the River Humber. The *Hull Daily Mail* put her photos in the newspaper repeatedly and pleaded for the public to come up with any clues. Radio Humberside and Yorkshire Television also did their best in publicising. Days went past without any news. Various agencies kept on appealing.

Soon after Teresa's disappearance, my brother-in-law, Prabha, who lives in London, his wife Grace, and her mother, Aunt Mary, came over and stayed with us. In a few days, dozens of relatives mainly from London, stayed over with us taking turns. My elder brother, working in Uganda, flew in and stayed for four weeks. There was a steady flow of the Kerala community from far and near visiting us daily, as was the custom back in Kerala and commonly in India, including many doctors and their wives. Mary was staying in bed most of the time. The ladies used to go straight to her. I felt a glimmer of relief to see that she was getting some emotional support.

Mary used to get very distressed after visits by Dr A, a lady consultant from Kerala working in the local NHS Trust, and Dr B, a GP who had a professional relationship with her. Dr A used to walk in like a guided missile into Mary's room, ignoring everybody and the surroundings, and used to see her as if performing some ritualistic healing. I was so engulfed looking after the children's schooling and liaising with police and other agencies on a daily basis. I could hardly get chance to talk to Mary in private since many relatives were with her all the time. Mary's close friends, Karen, Edna Hart and Lucy used to come every day and spend hours with her. Although I was in deep grief inside, I had to keep my composure outside to keep Mary and the children going and hoping and praying Teresa would return home. Since Dr B had a professional relationship with Mary, I kept updating him as the next of kin, when he came over. A friend of mine, an ex-police officer hinted to me that just relying on the sighting of the bike is sometimes misleading from his experience. So, we were living in hope all the time.

In the living room, it was mainly men. After a few days, the regular visitors from the Kerala community used my house as a workmen's club debating all current global affairs. Some of them used the occasion to give vivid picturesque descriptions advertising their new flashy cars, recent exotic holidays and some women joining in were going on about their latest design silk saris they bought after a shopping spree in Leicester. Overhearing these chit-chats, I felt nauseated; it was out of place and out of sense to show off pomp and glory in a house engulfed in profound grief and distress. I put up with all this because some sort of human presence and activities - good or bad was a welcome distraction to the black and deep eclipse of sorrow we were in. Also, my father used to tell me that if somebody comes to your home, even if it was your enemy, treat him with fairness, because he is your guest.

Karen kept on praying to St Antony to bring her back. On May 25th, 18 days after her disappearance, the police contacted me that a body of similar description to Teresa was spotted at Spurn Head. The devastating news hit our family. I had the most distressing and painful ordeal of my life – the formal process of identifying her. Looking into the ordeal of burial, there was no place in the Hessle Church cemetery. Karen came forward and said, "Teresa can sleep with me." She had a vacant plot in the cemetery which could accommodate three people.

The funeral was conducted on 2nd June at Our Lady of Lourdes Church, Hessle. Fr Michael O'Connor, who had been supporting us throughout the ordeal, conducted the ceremony. The church was packed. Teresa was laid to rest. The church collection £305.68, was donated to the Homeless & Rootless Project, as it was close to Teresa's heart.

14

Treachery and Betrayal

'I would rather be a little nobody, than to be an evil somebody.'

Abraham Lincoln

After Teresa's death, we were just managing to survive emotionally, mentally and financially. I had been off work for many weeks; all the expenses mounted up. Also, Thomas and Rowena were attending private school - Hymer's College. I started work and did some extra out of hours work to keep our heads above water. Dr A W Hussain and Dr S G Hussain, my partners at Anlaby Road Surgery were gracious, considerate and supportive.

Two weeks after the funeral, I received a letter from the General Medical Council stating that two doctors from Hull, both Indians, one from Kerala, from my own medical school (Dr A) and another, a GP (Dr B) had made complaints that I was not fit to practice. Dr A who had never set foot in my house for the previous 5 years or spoken to me even a full sentence, alleged that I was a heartless, uncaring man who did not care for his family. Having spoken just three sentences in the form of a banal "Hello" within the last 20 years, Dr A, a specialist, made slanderous statements about my personality, my 'conduct in India at my father-in-law's funeral' and many other malicious 'allegations' – an example of gross and grotesque abuse of power and position.

Dr B stated that 20 years back, while working in Nigeria, I was *raising money for my family* etc. He stated that he spoke to one of the doctors in India who treated me for 'depression long back in India' (I never knew such a thing happened, I would like to meet 'the phantom doctor'). Depression was portrayed like a heinous crime, especially by a GP who deals with so many depressed patients on a daily basis. Both of them started coming to my house only after Teresa's disappearance, along with nearly two dozen local doctor families. My house was full already with half a dozen relatives staying. There were also various personal allegations about my 'character'. They were not brave to make these complaints direct to the General Medical Council because they would have to give a sworn affidavit. Instead, they found a sneaky bypass and went to a health authority medical director, who, without visiting me or interviewing me or seeking opinion from the Local Medical Committee or my practice partners, channelled the complaints straight to the General Medical Council.

Especially being experienced doctors, they knew very well that we were in grief reaction. We were in a state of shock and numbing of emotions. A sense of frustration to surroundings and even in-animate objects set in. All sorts of emotions of loss, problems of life for the rest of the family and a multitude of worries about the future were capsizing all of us.

None of them had any working relationships with me, but they decided to act as 'judge and jury' to annihilate my professional competence. I learnt from reliable sources that there were conspiracy meetings between these two starting a week after Teresa's disappearance. While we were searching for our dear daughter, they were researching and fabricating 'evidence' to frame charges against me.

My legal team assessed both complaints and their findings were as follows:

1. Both complaints were dated the **same day**, 8th June 2001 (Teresa's funeral was on the 2nd June; so in a rush to finish me off also).
2. Both complaints were exactly **two-and-a-half pages** long.
3. Both complaints had **various common phrases**.

4. Both used official letterheads; Dr A had come in claiming as 'friend'. That *per se* was gross misuse of official position since there was no official role. Dr B had a professional relationship with Mary.

5. They cited family matters, which were outside the jurisdiction of the General Medical Council.

I presumed that they might have <u>cut and pasted</u> to save time, energy and paper. Dr A (from my medical school in India) might have had a score from yesteryears to settle. In the complaint, Dr A claimed as a 'close friend of the family'. But the reality was blatantly untrue; never set foot in my house previous five years since I was in financial hardship. Also, when Teresa applied to do four-weeks' work experience in that doctor's spouse's surgery, she was turned down with sudden rudeness, which upset her badly making her feel rejected.

In 1995, the Health Authority interviewed many candidates for the post of GP at Roos, Aldbrough and Burton-Pidsea. I was the successful one. Dr B was one among those interviewed. Shortly after, when he happened to see me casually at a medical meeting of GPs, he made it a point not to have any eye contact and avoided me at all costs while almost all GPs came forward, shook hands and congratulated me, because that was a covetable achievement. While I was surviving by doing out of hours work through a co-operative, Dr B tried to deprive my livelihood by pointing out that I was not a member of that co-operative.

Careful perusal of both the allegations showed that they were on a path of prejudice and collusion. Their ulterior motive was to, **derail mental equilibrium of a professional in grief reaction, professional homicide and disintegration of Abraham family** who were going through a horrible time after the death of Teresa, and not at all for the well-being my family or humanity. To achieve that goal, they were striking the iron when it was hot; exploiting a grieving, heart-broken and vulnerable lady as their tool in the name of 'emotional support'. None of these two 'ambassadors of the caring profession' had the basic courtesy to enquire how I was coping not even once. Dr A bearing a Christian name, broke the ninth commandment: 'You shalt not bear false witness against your neighbour'. I was a grieving father trying to exist in my own dwelling protecting my wife and children. Like hyenas targeting the weak and limping impala, they pounced, brutally exploiting the vulnerable state, with severe intrusions into my personal and family matters. They shrewdly manipulated a vulnerable lady to dig out marital issues out of context, which exist in every family (even the royal family was not exempt from their share of problems), which had no bearing on professional performance.

'Beware of false prophets, which come to you in sheep's clothing, but inwardly they are ravening wolves.'

Matthew 7:15

They cooked up hearsay stories. It was explicit that there was heinous collusion between the complainants which by itself was against the norms of justice, tilting the balance unfairly against the victim. I have strong work ethics and always practiced with the motto 'Do not take home to work; do not take work to home'.

The legal team observed that **personal vendetta, professional jealousy and exploitation of family tragedy** - the dreaded triad was executed with plumb precision to bring down a multi-talented and resourceful doctor, writer and medical school teacher so that the family would perish, by strangling the sole breadwinner of his livelihood. They were circling like vultures at the stench of death. To subject somebody going through grief reaction into a gruelling General Medical Council trial akin to a public court hearing was devilishly mean, since both the doctors knew very well their actions might cause financial hardship, social isolation and derail my mental equilibrium into an abyss precipitating self-harm or suicide. A survey showed 13 doctors committed suicide while undergoing GMC investigations in a span of four years. Dr Jane Wilcock from Salford, a GP of 20 years standing, described her experience when she was accused of professional misconduct. She became weepy, panicky and disconcertingly morbid for nine months until the GMC cleared her eventually.

I discussed subjecting these doctors to a 'lie detector test' with my legal team, which I would have done if I was not acquitted. I knew in the bottom of my heart that I would be cleared but I had to go through the formal process and wait.

Et tu, Brute?

Shakespeare, Julius Caesar

The last words of Julius Caesar, when he saw Brutus holding a dagger dripping with his blood, rang in my ears. Both doctors incited Mary to relive unpleasant matters of the past, knowing very well that would cause further damage to an already fragile woman in deep grief and resulting in chaos to disrupt the peace in the family.

The two doctors broke many of the universal rules governing the medical profession:

Hippocratic Oath - Whatever I see or hear in the lives of my patients, whether in connection with my professional practice or not, which ought not to be spoken of outside, I will keep secret, as considering all such things to be private.

Declaration of Geneva - I will respect the secrets that are confided in me, even after the patient has died; I will foster the honour and noble traditions of the medical profession; I will give to my teachers, colleagues, and students the respect and gratitude that is their due.

Breach of confidentiality – Dr B had a professional relationship with Mary. He had good inside knowledge which she disclosed, and was leaked out to others without her knowledge or consent. In 1997, a GP casually mentioned some medical details of a mutual patient to a dentist colleague during a round of golf; he was found guilty of serious professional misconduct by the General Medical Council and was suspended for six months.

Abuse of power and position - Dr A was a consultant and a lady from Kerala. Uninvited and unsolicited, she interviewed Mary and took notes without explanation and consent from her in my house and without my knowledge as her next of kin, abusing her specialist skills using techniques of coercion and persuasion. She was duty-bound to discuss with next of kin before even contemplating any such steps.

Breach of Human Rights Act- Article 8 of the European Convention on Human Rights provides a right to respect for one's 'private and family life, his home and his correspondence'. A consultant working in a local NHS Trust (public body), out of the blue, walked in uninvited and dug out intricate family affairs of bygone past most of it said to relate to life in India and Africa (outside UK jurisdiction) from a lady in the most vulnerable state of loss of her daughter, under duress. It was an act of severe intrusion into the privacy of my family, a blatant violation of the Human Rights Act.

Mens rea (**guilty mind**) is the mental element of a person's intention to commit a crime; or knowledge that one's action or lack of action would cause a crime to be committed. The person is morally and legally culpable. Dr A extracted intimate secrets of my family life, under the pretext of offering help and support.

There were only three people to support me. Dr Guy Clayton, GP from Beverley and Dr John Zacharias, GP from Scunthorpe and Dr Joseph Austin, GP from Bilton. They knew me well and gave all the support and encouragement. Then, my dad was behind me. I phoned him in India and briefed him about the situation. He replied, "In my working life in forests, I have dealt with so many animals who tried to destroy me. Not a snake has bit me; not an elephant has attacked me. A just man's son will come to no harm. Go fearless; God will be with you and speak for you and guide to safety."

The GMC hearing was at the London office. I went by train to London. While travelling, I envisaged the scenario of the GMC office, which I last visited in person in 1978, to hand over my registration documents. My vision was - the committee sat like judges on a magisterial bench with an ornamental mace looking down on the hapless creature trapped in the degrading dock. When I reached the scene, it was less hierarchical and appeared less intimidating than I thought.

The meeting started at 9 AM. I was read the letters of allegation by Drs A and B. The Medical Protection Society defence representative started the defence. Halfway through, I took over. I made it clear the hollowness of the fabricated allegations. I emphasised I was a grieving father in my home with my family and the motive was the disintegration of my family since I am the sole breadwinner, triggered by a personal vendetta and professional jealousy.

I submitted a folder containing all the publications I had written in the previous 7 years (94 in total) including the one in 1995, *General Practice 2020 Vision,* which was runner-up in the national competition. I made it explicit that I didn't want clemency (since I had not committed any offence) but I wanted justice. To me justice had to be meted out quickly because my job was the lifeline for my family. The meeting concluded by 1pm. I was advised to report back at 2. The role of the investigatory committee was to make sure the protection of patients, maintain confidence in the medical profession and uphold the standards expected of doctors.

I reported back at 2. I was told there were no charges against me and I was free to leave. It took only a few minutes. The ordeal was over. The hearing was fair. I had appeared as an expert witness in courts many times; but this was in sharp contrast since my reputation, personal values and career were being threatened.

The GMC followed *Audi alteram partem* ("listen to the other side"). It is the principle that no person should be judged without a fair hearing in which each party is given the opportunity to respond to the evidence against them. Within the common law system of justice, with its accusatorial procedure, the basic principle is that through conflict, truth emerges.

Justice delayed is justice denied. The GMC owes a **duty of care** to the medical profession. The law of the land has to prevail to protect the persecuted professional.

Lex est tutissima cassis; sub clypeo legis nemo decipitur

(Law is the safest helmet; under the shield of the law no one is deceived.)

Sir Edward Coke [1552-1634], great jurist of Jacobean era

On learning about the threat for my fitness to practice, so many respectable consultants wrote letters supporting me. My practice partner, Dr Aga Hussain, wrote: 'I have been practising for 41 years. He is one of the best partners I ever had. His sincerity, hard work and dedication have no limits… He is multi-talented. He is very popular among patients and the community in general... I am proud that he is my partner.'

My other practice partner Dr SG Hussain wrote: 'He has amicable manners and pleasant predisposition. He is very sincere, hardworking, flexible and understanding… His conduct is excellent personally and professionally.'

Dr Joseph Austin wrote: 'He has a very caring nature and I witnessed and appreciated his clinical acumen… He is extremely hardworking and conscientious, with very good rapport with patients... very caring and helpful. He is an excellent clinician… He is well thought of in the medical faculty and regularly contributes articles in medical journals.

Dr John Zacharias wrote: 'I have known him for over a decade. He has done locum work for our practice on many occasions. He is an outstanding clinician to whom no problem was too much to handle. He is at all times conscientious, caring and considerate.'

Most importantly, the Community Health Council was overwhelmed with an avalanche of letters of support from patients.

Mr E H, a retired ambulance man of 28 years' service: 'Both I and my wife cannot find fault with this doctor in any way. He has always treated us so much better than any other GP and we have the utmost confidence in him. I have some friends on his panel who say he is a very good doctor and a gentleman.'

Mr WW: 'I found Dr Abraham totally responsible, very sympathetic and caring; his conduct is very professional. All members of my family and close friends attending his surgery, speak very highly of his professionalism… I felt it was my duty to attend his daughter's internment… the church was packed to capacity… a tribute to his standing in the community…'

Mr PG: 'I have lived in Hull 45 years… He is the best doctor I have come across. Patients treated by him say that he is a doctor of high quality and fine manners. The whole community in Hull speaks very highly about him.'

Mr JB: 'He is the best doctor we had… He is hardworking, he used to work 15 hours a day… he is highly talented… he has admirable manners and high professional standards.'

So many more patients and members of the public came forward. I wish to express my deep gratitude to each and every one who supported me in the darkest time of my life and career.

I tried to analyse why human beings try to harm another one in this way. The answer is probably jealousy (/ˈdʒɛləs)- feeling or showing an envious resentment of someone or their achievements, possessions, or perceived advantages.

'Beware of jealousy, my lord! It's a green-eyed monster that makes fun of the victims it devours'.

Shakespeare, Othello, Act 3, Scene 3

Possible reasons were:

- I got the rural practice in 1995, while Dr B was not successful at the interview.
- I had won £3000 prescribing incentive.
- Every third week, I was in the press; I had 94 publications from 1994 to 2000, which was well beyond imagination. I had been the 'Voice of Hull' for the medical profession on the national scene.
- In 1995, my article on '2020 Vision of General Practice' won national acclaim.
- I was a tutor at Leeds Medical School.
- I was invited for a meeting with the Head of Primary care, NHS, in London.
- I had an audience with Pope John Paul.
- I had met Nobel laureate Archbishop Desmond Tutu.

All these were in the press. I got involved in so many other public commitments. All these, I achieved by sheer hard work and dedication.

'Falsehood flies, and truth comes limping after it, so that when men come to be undeceived, it is too late; the jest is over, and the tale hath had its effect.'

Jonathan Swift (1667-1745)

15

Cricket

'Cricket – it is more than a game. It is an institution.'

Thomas Hughes

The TV presenter and comedy writer, Denis Norden, once commented, 'It is a funny kind of month, October. For the really keen cricket fans, it is when you realise that your wife left you in May'. In most sports, the role of captain is not terribly demanding or stressful. For example, in football, his role is to smile and toss the coin, speak to the press after the match and act as intermediary between the players and the management. But captaining a cricket team is one of the most daunting and demanding tasks in sport. Apart from the jobs mentioned, he has to be the motivator, man-manager, mathematician, weather forecaster, selector and psychologist and so on.

Cricket is a funny old game. About 130 years back, one of the great players W G Grace (Grace Gates at Lords) was playing in Hull, he hit the ball 37 miles!! Amazing!

Well, he smashed the ball into a passing railway truck and next stop was Leeds. In Adelaide, during a Test Match, an extra fielder sustained a fractured leg and denied England 2 runs; a powerful shot was on the way to boundary but a seagull intercepted and the ball came to a grinding halt. 1979 Australia v England Test Match: The score board read - *Lillee c Willey b Dilley 19;* it was a coincidental rhyming.

In 1990, Mrs Margaret Thatcher, used cricket as a metaphor of her life, when she made a speech at the Lord Mayor's Banquet. Her opening remarks were, "Since I first went in to bat 11 years ago." If I use her analogy - when I first went in to bat 30 years ago, cricket was mainly played as Test Matches by a handful of countries. Slowly and steadily the infectious enthusiasm spread across the globe. Now, cricket is played in **125** countries -(10 full members, 38 associate and 59 affiliate) and in 3 main formats.

Also, when I started listening to Test Matches, the pocket transistor was the main gadget. Now, with the advent of high tech transmission, cricket is seen live on all corners of the earth.

Village Cricket - in spite of all the glamour and glory of modern cricket, let us not forget the humble beginning of cricket in the village of Hambledon in Hampshire. Village cricket is like homemade brew. Lush-green field, the backdrop of a Gothic parish church and local pub, usually adjacent to a canal or duck pond. The other accompaniments are - rudimentary black score board with white letters, often rattling in the wind, deck of easy chairs for the gentlemen who often chain-smoke their pipes, picnic tables with assortment of crisps, sandwiches and multi-coloured drinks, row of rugs where the team members' wives and girlfriends try to swing or bowl bouncers by exhibiting their curves. After the match, winners, losers and part of the crowd migrate to the local pub to put the finishing touches to the day. Village cricket is really mesmerising.

Some of the facets of cricket are quite fascinating and intriguing:

Olympics- Can you believe? Great Britain is the ever-reigning Olympic champion in cricket. In the 1900 Paris Olympics, there were only 4 teams competing. Belgium and Holland withdrew. So it was GB v France and it was easily won by Team GB. Well, the French team was mainly staff from the British embassy. That was it; cricket has never been an Olympic game since then.

Runs - cricket is **all about runs**; all are **running** all the time. Everybody knows Brian Lara's 400 not out, Sachin Tendulkar holding highest runs in test and ODI and 100 centuries, but many do not remember how many wickets Muralitharan and Shane Warne took, and who holds the record for catches. Maybe the justification is that the batsman may get out on the first ball, while the bowler can keep on bowling. The great West Indian Garry Sobers was the first batsman to hit six sixes in an over. Nottinghamshire v Glamorgan. The bowler was Malcom Nash. After the match, Garry was having a drink in the corridor. He saw Nash coming towards him but pretended to look out through the window, thinking Nash might be angry with him for hitting him all over the park. Nash came and tapped Sobers on his shoulder with a smile and said, "Garry, you are not the only one to go into the record book; I also got in with you."

English actor Oliver Reed once commented, "I suppose doing a love scene with Raquel Welch roughly corresponds to scoring a century before lunch." On the other hand, if you are out first ball, as cricket writer JM Barrie put it – "Pretend you only came out for the fun of it; go and sit by yourself near the hedge."

Sledging - sledging has become a side dish in cricket. If we hold an International Sledging Competition, Australia will be the outright winner. But all nations try their part. Sledging comes with varying pace and from different angles; just to give some examples - Fred Truman was bowling; first slip Subba Row missed the catch - the ball went between his legs.

SR apologised. "I should have kept my legs together, Fred."

Truman turned to him and said, "Not you, son; your mother should have."

Jeff Thompson, the Australian fast bowler who used to terrorise batsmen, once said, "Stiff upper lip; let us see how stiff it is, when it is split."

Rodney Marsh (Australian w/k) to Ian Botham, "How is your wife, and <u>my</u> kids?"

1991 Adelaide Test Pakistan v Australia - while batting, Javed Miandad called Merv Hughes a "fat bus conductor". A bit later when Javed got out, Merv shouted, "Tickets, please." Thus, the sledging game goes on and on!

Boredom - in contrast to the fast-moving T20 and ODIs, in Test Matches, at times, the passages of play can be dull and dragging. It is the commentators' role to keep the crowd awake. One of the illustrious and hilarious commentators was Brian Johnston. To pick some of his words – "Neil Harvey is at first slip, with his legs apart, waiting for a tickle." In another match, he said, "This bowler is like my dog; three short legs and balls that swing each way."

Cricket is not complete without the sense of humour of the commentators. They add the spice to the meals.

Crowd - without the crowd, cricket is a dull and dry game. Crowds support their teams patriotically and passionately. Sometimes they get too excited and take clothes off, streaking! Famous Australian commentator Richie Benaud witnessed an episode when a streaker made a high jump over the wicket knocking the bails off. He commented, "There was a slight interruption for athletics."

England v Australia - an Australian banner read "England will win if Camilla Parker bowls."

India v Australia, Sydney – A banner read, 'If you want to commit robbery, do it now because God is watching Sachin Tendulkar batting.'

Spirit of Cricket - Cricketer's Bible Tom Smith summarises it nicely. "Cricket is a game that owes much of its unique appeal to the fact it should be played not only within its laws, but also within the Spirit of the Game." This speaks for itself.

In the summer of 2004, I organised a cricket match **GPs** v **Consultants** at the Police Sports club, Hull. It was a sunny and dry day, with a clear blue sky, ideal for play. The Consultants' team captain, Dr Mathew, won the toss and elected to bat. They put up a challenging total of 159. I opened the batting for GPs. I was out for 18. Soon there was a collapse; we were 93 for 9. We were written off and staring at defeat. Being the captain, I became that restless and started pacing outside the boundary rope shouting to our last pair various motivating words. Dr Colin Fairhurst did a fantastic knock, virtually 'batting at both ends' and we won against all odds. We managed to grab victory from the jaws of defeat. It was a typical example of the glorious uncertainties of cricket. (Or was it due to Captain Courageous?)

I used to umpire in the East Yorkshire cricket league for about 10 years. When I stood in the middle wearing the white coat, I kept telling myself that I was the judge in this game of gentlemen. The major global sport of football is not considered gentlemanly due to the monotonously repeated scenario of scantily clad sweaty young men kissing and cuddling each other in public after each goal. As per the laws, the umpires are the sole judges of fair and unfair play. To stand still, a singular and solitary man carrying an unbelievable burden of frustrating responsibilities, was a challenge to the nervous system. Predicting the gist of every delivery with mathematical precision and certainty gave an aura of intermingled pleasure and pain. At times, I had to be the pentagon of protection for the batsman from being harassed or cajoled.

The ground with lush green grass, partially bordered by trees under a wide iridescent cloud-free blue sky in summer, a quiet timelessness which was indigenously and quintessentially English - all depicted a pastoral beauty to the game. Unlike any other sports, the game preys on doubt. There is only one thing in everybody's mind - THE NEXT BALL. Until it is delivered all are in suspense. At times, when the scarce makeshift scorer was ensconced at comfortable vantage point, I had to encode the message and attach it to the legs of a pigeon flying past that cooed away and wait for the decoded message to transmit back.

After the match, we all retired for customary drinks. Facts, fiction and gossip - all went up in the air interspersed with cigarette smoke producing a misty whirlwind. I could see various eagle eyes sparkling. Restricting myself to basic friendly gestures, I stayed poker-faced, downed the drink and resisted making any inflammatory pronouncements. My co-umpires were wonderful, supportive and imaginative. They offered timely tips.

The lingering loveliness of moments caught in the infectious enthusiasm of the leather ball with cross stripes and golden letters whizzing past, stumps flying, the puck noise of willow hitting the ball, fielders chasing around in frenzy and the vacant gaze of fieldsmen when lofted for six, the proud lean of the batsman over the baton scoring boundary, the lion-roar of the bowler having taken a wicket and midwicket celebratory congregation - all make up the great game.

As Sir Pelham Warner remarked, "The very word cricket has become a synonym for all that is true and honest. To say 'that is not cricket' implies something underhand; something not in keeping with the best ideals." To commence the proceedings holding aloft the cherry red ball, the 'British sphere of influence' in the Rolls Royce of all sports as the Master of Ceremony, lively outside albeit lonely inside, is of great pride and privilege.

*   *   *

2014 - RIP Philip Hughes

In 2009, I was in London for a few days. A friend of mine took me to Middlesex, his home county's game. I saw Philip Hughes playing. I commented to my friend, "He is the Australian with a bit of David Gower in him." Indeed, he was a stylish enigmatic batsman. In November 2014, playing in a Sheffield Shield match at Sydney, Sean Abbott bowled a 90 miles per hour bouncer which hit Hughes on head, tore the vertebral artery and his time on earth came to an end. As a lover of cricket and humanity, it devastated me. In my early playing days at medical school, I also was hit on the head but luckily escaped any serious injury. The global cricketing world paid glorious tributes after his untimely death.

In June 2016, Shivil Kaushik, an Indian Premier League cricketer playing for the team, Gujarat Lions, was arranged to play for Hull. He stayed with me for the period of contract for 3 months. He was a slow left arm chinaman bowler with a unique action resembling Paul Adams of South Africa. It was his first outing outside India. Being my guest, I looked after him very well. He enjoyed his tenure and went back to India after a successful season.

16

Military Work

'A true soldier fights not because he hates what is in front of him, but because he loves what is behind him.'

G K Chesterton

In 2003, I got a request to do three weeks work at an RAF station in Lincoln. I was aware of the formidable military bible, King's Regulations that one of the commonest charges to bring an officer to Court Martial is for 'behaviour unbecoming of an officer and a gentleman'. Although being a civilian doctor, it did not affect me directly, I was aware of my code of conduct. The station liked me and I liked the station. So I ended up working there for 18 months. I took additional qualifications in aviation medicine and continued to serve the RAF at various stations.

Germany

Working with BFG (British Forces in Germany) was a memorable and pleasant passage of time. I have worked at various stations - Munster, Paderborn, Fallingbostel, Ramstein, just to name a few.

The weekends were free. I used to take the *Schones-Wochenende-Ticket* (Happy weekend Ticket) and set off in the morning and return in the night. This was a day pass for a party of up to five people for 37 Euros, putting our rail fares to shame. The Inter-city *Deutsche Bahn* are semi-fast at 150mph while *Thalys* high speed trains are at 186mph. Although driving on an Autobahn is faster than our motorways, accidents are less frequent comparatively.

Rhine River cruise was a prime attraction. There were a series of castles along the banks of the Rhine. There are lots of vineyards on banks off Rhine. I went for a wine-tasting masterclass in Koblenz.

It should be about one-third full. Loosely follow these steps to evaluate the wine visually. First, look straight down into the glass, then hold the glass to the light, and finally, give it a tilt, so the wine rolls over. Viewing the wine through the side of the glass held in light shows you how clear it is, its edges. This will allow you to see the wine's complete colour range, not just the dark centre. Tilting the glass so the wine thins out toward the rim will provide clues to the wine's age and weight. Finally, give the glass a good swirl. You can swirl it most easily by keeping it firmly on a flat surface; open air 'freestyle' swirling is not recommended for beginners. Note if the wine forms 'legs' or 'tears' that run down the sides of the glass. Wines that have good legs are wines with more alcohol and glycerine content, which generally indicates that they are bigger, riper, more mouth-filling and denser than those that do not.

Take a good sniff, give the glass a swirl, but don't bury your nose inside it. Instead, you want to hover over the top like a helicopter pilot surveying rush hour traffic. Take a series of quick, short sniffs, then step away and let the information filter through to your brain. Take a sip, not a large swallow, of wine into your mouth and try sucking on it as if pulling it through a straw. This aerates the wine and circulates it throughout your mouth. A complete wine is balanced, harmonious, complex and evolved, with a lingering, satisfying finish.

*   *   *

I visited my cousin, Fr James, who had been a parish priest in Nuremberg for the last 20 years. Nuremburg is the second largest city in the federal state of Bavaria. The Kaiserberg castle was built in 1040 by the German King Henry III, who went to become The Holy Roman Emperor.

The city bears the painful ugly scars of the brutal Nazi regime. Zeppelin Field was the Nazi party's rally ground. After World War II, in 1945-46, the Allied Forces conducted the military tribunals according to International Law - The Nuremberg Trials.

*   *   *

In 2007 at RAF Leeming, I met Europe's oldest man, Henry Allingham aged 111, who was the last surviving member of the Royal Naval Air Service. As an air mechanic with the **Royal Naval** Air Service (RNAS), in 1916 Allingham witnessed the battle of Jutland from the decks of *HMS Kingfisher* in the North Sea, and was the last survivor of either side. He also saw at first hand, often under fire, the horrors of Flanders, at one point nearly drowning in a shell hole full of decaying bodies in Passchendaele.

In 2006, he went to Germany to meet Robert Meier, who was 109. They were wheeled side-by-side to lay a wreath on the local war memorial. Then the two men, who had been foes in the same sector of Ypres, shook hands with great tenderness. They were the two oldest men in their respective countries. Henry had seen W G Grace at the Oval while Robert had met the Kaiser.

I took inspiration from Henry's words. "I had two breakdowns both when trying to do the work of three men. The trick is to look after yourself and know your limitations." I was moved by his vitality, dignity and humour, for he had an irrepressible spirit. In his later years, he felt he must speak of the war in order not to forget the sacrifice of so many young men. "There's a lot I've tried hard to forget. I've got a lot to be thankful for. I've had a unique sort of life. I've scraped the barrel and I've had the cream." Henry William Allingham, born 6 June 1896, died 18 July 2009. RIP.

*   *   *

On a number of occasions, I worked at RAF Scampton which is the home of the Red Arrows, officially known as the Royal Air Force Aerobatic Team. The team was formed in late 1964 as an all-RAF team, replacing a number of unofficial teams that had been sponsored by RAF commands. The Red Arrows have a prominent place in British popular culture, with their aerobatic displays a fixture of British summer events. The badge of the Red Arrows shows the aircraft in their trademark diamond nine formation, with the motto *Éclat*, a French word meaning 'brilliance' or 'excellence'.

Initially, they were equipped with seven Folland Gnat trainers inherited from the RAF Yellowjacks display team. This aircraft was chosen because it was less expensive to operate than front-line fighters. In their first season, they flew at 65 shows across Europe. In 1966, the team was increased to nine members, enabling them to develop their Diamond Nine formation. In late 1979, they switched to the BAE Hawk trainer. The Red Arrows have performed over 4,800 displays in 57 countries worldwide.

While I was working there, Suryakiran (The Rays of Sun), the Indian Air Force Aerobatic Team, came over for an exchange visit and training. The team composes of nine aircraft formation, flying the indigenously built

Kiran MKII aircrafts. They are the ambassadors of India and the Indian Air Force, taking immense pride in showcasing the highest standards of traditions. The teamwork, professionalism and confidence are the hallmarks of the team. *E'spirit de corps* and absolute discipline are the motivating force in the team's quest for excellence in each and every display. The team strives hard and continues to maintain excellent standard in precision Formation aircraft flying living up to the motto of the Squadron 'Always the Best'.

*   *   *

The poppy is close to the heart and people wear it close to the heart near the left pocket. In 2009, I paid respect to Remembrance Day by writing an article on the poppy in the publication, **PULSE,** 'Lest we forget: poppy's role in history of medicine.'

From time immemorial, human life has been associated with the poppy. Celebrating Remembrance Day brings a timely, poignant and painful reminder of its significance. The Greek depicted Hypnos (sleep), Nyx (night) and Thanatos (death) wreathed in poppies. Poppies were ornamental on the statues of Apollo, Aesculapius, Aphrodite, Pluto and Demeter. When Pluto abducted Persephone, the daughter of Demeter, he ate poppies to fall asleep and forget the grief. The poppy was considered magical as well as poisonous and was used in various religious ceremonies.

Hippocrates (460-377 BC) made various references to the poppy in many medicinal potions. He distinguished between red, white and black poppies and was aware of the therapeutic effects of unripe, ripe and baked varieties. He mentioned poppy juice as hypnotic, styptic and cathartic. Herakleides of Pontus(340 B C) mentioned the poppy as a means of euthanasia - 'Since the population lives to a ripe old age, they do not wait until they are very old for death to take them, but take themselves out of life, some by means of poppy, others with hemlock.' Celsus (First century AD) referred to the poppy as a painkiller, hypnotic and antidote. Galen (second century AD) mentioned, 'Opium is the strongest of the drugs which numb the senses and induces a deadening sleep.'

Shakespeare was well aware of the medicinal effects of the poppy:

'Not poppy nor mandragora, not all the drowsy syrups of the world,

Shall ever medicine thee to that sweet sleep, which thou owe'st yesterday.'

Othello, III, 334

Poppies grow in conditions of disturbed earth. In the early 19th century, the Napoleonic Wars transformed bare land into a refuse tip of dead soldiers; poppies thrived there like fieldfare. In the First World War, some of the fiercest fighting occurred in the Flanders and Picardy regions of Belgium and Northern France. After the mayhem, the fields were filled with floods of poppies. In 1918, John McCrae, a doctor serving with the Canadian Armed Forces, was deeply touched with the trail of devastation he saw and wrote the poem:

In Flanders Fields

In Flanders fields the poppies blow,

Between the crosses, row on row,

That mark our place; and the sky

The larks, still bravely singing, fly

Scarce heard amid the guns below.

We are the dead. Short days ago

We lived, felt dawn, saw sunset glow,

Loved, and were loved, and now we lie

In Flanders Fields.

Take up our quarrel with the foe:

To you from falling hands we throw

The torch; be yours to hold it high.

If ye break faith with us who die

We shall not sleep, though poppies grow

In Flanders Fields.

On the 11th hour of the 11th day of the 11th month of 1918, the First World War ended. The poppy became a lasting symbol for the fallen heroes. American war secretary, Miona Michael, inspired by McCrae's poem, started selling poppies to raise money for the ex-service community. The first official British Legion Poppy day was held on 11 November 1921. Since then, Poppy Appeal has become a solemn ingredient in our national calendar. In 1922, The Poppy Factory was founded in Richmond, Surrey. In 1933, white poppy was introduced by women's Co-operative Guild, as a symbol of peace and end to all wars. But the British Legion did not approve of this and the initiative met premature extinction.

Poppy (*Papaver somniferum*) is an annual flower growing on a central pod. On scratching, the pod oozes out milky latex called opium. From this, opiates like codeine and morphine are derived, which are extensively used in daily medical practice. Thus, the poppy, which thrived from the blood, tears and sweat of fallen heroes, is being used to alleviate the suffering of all of us.

*   *   *

I had the opportunity to work at RAF Northolt on a few occasions. That is where the most memorable words of Winston Churchill were uttered on 20 August 1940, about the RAF personnel – 'Never in the field of human conflict was so much owed by so many to so few.'

One of the sad chapters of working as doctor in the armed forces is witnessing the sordid plight of young men and women returning from the theatres of active conflict abroad, returning with horrific injuries including loss of limbs. A young man running around playing football yesterday has been crippled to a wheelchair for the rest of his life overnight - the cruel irony of fate. I have been intrigued by the bizarre and perplexing compensation pattern. There has been perineal problems in compensation for those personnel who sustain severe injuries in the line of duty. The

Daily Mail, 8 March 2014, reported 'Lance Bombardier Ben Parkinson, 23, was blown up by a mine in 2006 in Afghanistan. He was left in a coma for months, sustained 37 injuries, including loss of both legs, damage to skull, spine and pelvis. He was offered £152,000 in compensation. After his mother's persistence and public outcry, he was awarded £570,000.

I have enjoyed working in the military environment and did my best. When I left St George Barracks, North Luffenham in 2012, the commanding officer wrote to me. 'The contribution you have made in such a limited period of time is truly noteworthy and I can say without doubt that you leave the regiment in a better place than you found it.'

*   *   *

When I was working at RAF Lossiemouth, I went on a guided tour of Glen Moray Distillery, in Elgin.

Whisky is an integral part of Scottish life. It is the main drink at weddings and *deoch an dorius* (final door drink) to any guest leaving a party. It is the drink de riguer at every funeral of the rich and poor alike. As mentioned in Humphry Clinker, whisky was given 'with great success to infants, as a cordial, in the confluent smallpox'. In 1822, when King George IV visited Scotland, he enjoyed Glenlivet whisky. The only drink Queen Victoria liked was whisky.

Glen Moray is a single malt whisky distilled on the banks of the River Lossie since 1897, just outside Elgin. In its long history, the award-winning Glen Moray has been distilled in time-honoured fashion, by hand, never rushed or forced, always in balance, steady and with care, round the clock, seven days a week. In its lifetime, the distillery has known only 5 distillery managers. Know-how, myths and trade secrets passed through the generations to ensure every drop has the same light character as the last. Glen Moray Classic is fresh on the nose, with aroma of barley, wet grass and gentle fruit notes. The palate is balanced and mild with a taste of nuts, citrus fruit and oak.

17

2005 - Turbulent Year

'In the midst of turbulence, we hang on to hope.'

Lailah Akita

Hyde Six Trial

The six doctors who signed the second part of cremation forms done by Dr Harold Shipman, were put on trial by the General Medical Council. Seeing their plight, I fought for them in the national publication *GP*, in January 2005.

'The GMC hearing undergone by the six GPs who signed forms C at Shipman's request, is an affront to the collective *conscience of general practice.* In the first place, how can a doctor find out about mortality in a colleague's practice?

Serious professional misconduct has been defined as conduct that "would reasonably be regarded as disgraceful or dishonourable by his professional brethren of good repute and standing". As Manchester

LMC secretary Dr Peter Fink stated, "Their practice was no better or worse than their colleagues' across the country."

'Furthermore, '...a doctor is not negligent if he acts in accordance with a practice accepted at the time as proper by a responsible body of medical opinion.' (Bolam v Frein Hospital Management Committee [1957] 2 AIIER 118. If this test is applied, either these doctors pass or all 33,000 GPs should face GMC hearings. At the end, all of them were acquitted.

*   *   *

Pope John Paul's Funeral

The most important event I attended in my lifetime was the funeral of Pope John Paul II. *All roads lead to Rome*; the adage proved right. Four million people flocked to Rome to pay their final respects. The outpouring of grief and sense of loss appeared a worldwide phenomenon. The Vatican Curia went into overdrive almost to crashing point about the infinitesimal logistics of finding order to the land and air traffic, provision of water, sanitation and medical care for those who descended into Rome. About 18000 people per hour passed the body of the pope lying in state for five days. I went with my wife Mary and son

Thomas. When we reached the body, the Italian Police made a loud order, "No movement." US President Bush, wife Laura Bush, Senior Bush and Bill Clinton walked in, knelt beside the body, prayed and left. Then we were allowed to proceed.

Serpentine queues stretched over River Tiber and the cobble-stone piazzas overlooked by majestic palazzos with sculptures by Bernini and Michelangelo. The angels and saints on the frescoed ceilings peeped through the windows to have a sneak preview of the colossal multitude of mankind turning out to see the 'People's Pope'. Vatican, the smallest country in the world, received the whole world. St Peter's Basilica, the matrix of churches, with its mighty silver-blue dome blending into the sky, gave a sense of gazing into the infinity. The symmetrical semi-circular wings of the graceful colonnade appeared as outstretched arms receiving the whole of mankind with a universal embrace.

The open-air funeral mass was conducted in St Peter's Square. The UN Secretary General, the British Prime Minister, Prince Charles, three successive US presidents, five kings, seven queens, scores of presidents and world leaders were flanked by 300,000 people in the square and millions outside. The flags waving of various countries by men, women and children of all ages and nationalities gave an impression of a United Nations meeting. After buying an air ticket with his whole year's salary, Kyrian Atugo, 27, a civil servant from Nigeria, remarked, "He is the President of the World". By going to meet the man who tried to assassinate him, in the prison cell and forgiving him, the pope illustrated to the world the lesson of forgiveness, peace and reconciliation. It was poignant that the message permeated over his dead body - leaders at war who never spoke to each other shook hands and embraced.

The widely popular telegenic Pope John Paul II had phenomenal charisma and was a global communicator. 'The Pilgrim Pope' travelled to 129 countries reaching out to the masses, clocking air miles 30 times encircling the globe or 3 times trip to the moon. The millions repaid him by travelling from every corner of earth to say goodbye. His death brought together different worlds - ancient and modern, secular and spiritual, believers and non-believers. Rome ran out of tissues and dark glasses; even many dignitaries could not prevent tears at the ceremony.

The spectacular Roman sunshine lasted for six days so that the masses were not inconvenienced. Two hours after the funeral, dark clouds loomed over the skies, a series of thunder and lightning followed; nature's way of giving the 21-gun salute to the great man. Soon the heavens opened symbolising the cry of mother earth lasting for almost a day- and-a-half.

John Paul II was a man of firm faith who withstood the weight of the Pontificate and steered the rudder of St Peter's bark without fear or favour. He was humane in manners, firm in doctrine and had a balanced attitude. To the world, he was the very embodiment of democracy, social justice and above all champion of human dignity. Aptly, the world turned out in colossal numbers to pay homage to the world statesman.

$*$ $*$ $*$

Father's Death:

In 2005, shortly after the pope's death, my father died at home aged 86, in India. I fixed the funeral for the next week so that all necessary arrangements could be made, and also allowing time for me to make adjustments here. I went with Mary and Thomas; the flight landed at Cochin at 10.30am. We reached home by 1.30 in the afternoon.

The funeral procession started from my home to the local church at Pacha which was less than a mile away. The entire village, almost all relatives, friends and ex-colleagues, making up a total of over a thousand people walked slowly and serenely behind the funeral cortege. Leading the procession was a cross and black ceremonious umbrella followed by other paraphernalia of pictures of various saints. The highlight was the band-set singing the funeral songs, which are sung in such a way that even the stone-hearted would end up wiping tears. The church ceremony was conducted by Archbishop Joseph Powathil. The weather was kind in remaining dry and sunny. My dad was laid to rest.

18

2006 - Hectic Times

'Beware the barrenness of a busy life.'

Socrates

There was widespread coverage in the press about Liberal Democrat Leader, Rt Hon Charles Kennedy's alcohol problem. There were also reference to the same issue in medical world. I wrote to him offering my sincere support. He replied to me in Feb 2016: 'I have been deeply touched by people who have been generous enough to take time and trouble to make contact in similar fashion... I remain positively determined to maintain my active participation in public life, encouraged hugely by the wave of goodwill expressed in recent times to myself and my family. My great gratitude to you again for getting in touch.'

From time immemorial, alcohol has been part of human society. In the wedding of Cana of Galilee, Jesus converted six jars each containing 30 gallons water into wine (John 2:3-11).

'Go, eat your food with gladness, and drink your wine with a joyful heart, for God has already approved what you do.' - Ecclesiastes 9:7

Alcohol is a stimulant, social lubricant, food and fuel. In the UK, 89 percent of the adult population (9 out of 10) drink alcohol. The practice is widely normal and socially acceptable. Any occasion - whether social, religious, wedding etc – is marked invariably by vast amounts of alcohol being served. The eating out culture indirectly increases alcohol consumption. The introduction of children's certificates for public houses in England and Wales had attracted more families.

The alcohol industry is very powerful. In the UK, about one million people are employed in alcohol-related industries. In England and Wales, there is a public house for every 550 people. The alcoholic drinks market is worth £25 billion per annum. Taxation on alcohol is an important source of income for the government, totalling five percent of national income. Most major breweries sponsor sporting events. An open European market in 1992 has compounded the difficulties in dealing with the alcohol problem. The World Health Organisation Declaration in Alma Atta (1978) proposed target for reduction of alcohol by 25% by 2000. But alcohol consumption in the UK has doubled up in the past 30 years.

In the **Health of the Nation** document, alcohol was included as a key target. But having done that, government increased the opening hours of public houses. On a national basis, the government should make a commitment to curb and counter the rise of alcohol consumption in order to reduce alcohol-related illnesses. Public awareness needs to be increased. The campaign about 'sensible' drinking produces a smokescreen since most people think they drink 'sensibly'. Local communities have untapped resources. A campaign in Thunder Bay, Canada, has shown that the perception and enthusiasm of local communities hold the key in managing the sale and use of alcohol. Most health professionals and MPs drink in a responsible way.

*   *   *

March 2006 - Sir Roy Meadow

I wrote in the publication, *DOCTOR*, when the high court overturned the GMC's decision to strike off Prof Sir Roy Meadow, as a victory for justice. Prof Roy Meadow, internationally renowned paediatrician, acting as an expert witness in the trial of Sally Clark, made one mistake of misinterpreting and misunderstanding the statistics. The GMC panel admitted that it was a mistake that was easily and widely made. Yet, in the politically correct climate, the GMC in its wisdom thought it is better to strike Prof Meadow off. Putting passion before reason in this brutal attack, meant the world would have been deprived of such an eminent doctor.

Though capital punishment was abolished by the parliament, the GMC tends to use its own version of professional annihilation of doctors, their reputation and livelihoods too frequently. Prof Meadow's career was destined premature death. As Lazarus was given reprieve from the grave, the high court gave him a new lease of life. Presiding over, Justice Collins said, 'It may be proper to have criticised him for not disclosing his lack of expertise, but that does not justify a finding of serious professional misconduct.'

The keystone of the main arch of legal system is that justice must be seen to be done. The legal foundation of this was laid in the constitutional case Scott v Scott (1913) AC 417, in which Lord Halsbury said, 'Every court in the land is open to every subject of the King.'

*   *   *

September - Meeting the Man of 'Hope'

I had an audience with William Jefferson Clinton, 42nd President of the USA, in September 2006, when he came to give a lecture on leadership. I took Mary and Thomas with me. Also, I flew my daughter Rowena from St Andrews to meet him. The meeting venue could not have been more appropriate; at the Royal Albert Hall in South Kensington, London, which is one of the most treasured and distinctive buildings in the UK. It is held in trust for the nation and managed by a registered charity. It was opened in 1871, ten years after the death of Prince Albert due to Typhoid Fever. The hall can seat about 5,200. As I rushed towards this iconic and versatile building, the striking giant dome reminded me of Queen Victoria's words during the construction, when Her Majesty visited the Hall. Seeing the vast wedding-cake like structure, the comment was, 'It looks like the British constitution'. Granville's letter to Lord Canning mentioned it 'the eighth wonder of the world'.

President Clinton spoke regarding the fundamental nature of the 21st century which was marked by (a) globalisation enhanced by travel, trade and immigration (b) independence; he highlighted the traditional economic co-operation between The United States and Europe. (c) Unequal, unstable and unsustainable world; unequal distribution of resources - it is a matter of universal shame that two-and-a-half billion people exist without proper sanitation. Malaria and AIDS have been causing significant morbidity and mortality in nearly one-fifth of Africa's population. The conflicts and wars are making the world unstable. The world is getting more unsustainable due to global warming and finite sources of energy.

For every problem, there is a solution. He suggested the measures to make world a better place: (a) integration of communities at local, regional and national levels (b) equal opportunities by shared responsibilities and creating a sense of belonging (c) better safety and security by reducing tension due to conflicts by dialogue, reduction of weapons of mass destruction (which he called MAD - Mutually Assisted Destruction) and reduction of global warming (d) building more co-operative institutions and (e) home improvements on a global scale.

The *modus operandi* to take up these challenging roles by governments, non-governmental organisations and most importantly by each and every one of us to make a contribution to the well-being of the world. The Clinton foundation has been actively involved in the reduction of poverty, treatment of HIV and AIDS and global warming reduction. He insisted that we must set examples to our future generations. He remarked, 'Those among us who bring successful changes are the economic guerrillas.' He recalled the greatest world leader he has met, Nelson Mandela, whose mind was in a state of freedom while his body was in captivity.

The body and blend of his speech permeated an aura of inspirational grandeur. The master magician drew everybody in with his radiant smile and magnetic eyes. Everybody felt stunned by the great telegenic talisman. He exhibited the serenity of an actor who memorised his script well and mesmerised the audience. At the end, the gathering gave a standing ovation producing a man-made thunder which resonated a thousand times in the great hall of fame. It was almost reminiscent of the deafening noise when a shell hit the dome of the Royal Albert Hall in 1917.

Vini, Vidi, Vici (I came, I saw, I conquered) - Julius Caesar's words were apt to be applied there. Since

Clara Butt sang 'Land of Hope and Glory' in that hall in 1914, nobody else had whipped up passions and frenzies of an audience until Clinton did it that day. The great global communicator won the hearts and minds of us all. It was a quixotic experience to see the man who played a major role in reshaping the world. Bill Clinton was born in a town called Hope, Arkansas. Yes, he did kindle the candle of hope in a glorious style!

*   *   *

'Hull, Hell and Halifax.'

Thomas got admission to St Matthew's University, Cayman Islands. In 2004, I went with him to oversee the induction. Cayman Islands, a British Overseas Territory, encompasses three islands in the western Caribbean Sea. Grand Cayman, the largest island, is known for its beach resorts and varied scuba diving and snorkelling sites. Cayman Brac is a popular launch point for deep-sea fishing excursions. Little Cayman, the smallest island, is home to diverse wildlife, from endangered iguanas to seabirds such as red-footed boobies.

Hell is a group of short, black, limestone formations located in Grand Cayman, Located in West Bay, it is roughly the size of half a football field. Visitors are not permitted to walk on the limestone formations but viewing platforms are provided. There is a post office with long queues all the time since all tourists want to send postcard from Hell. I also sent many cards to friends saying, 'To you on earth, with regards from Hell'. So, I have been to all the three important places - Hull, Hell and Halifax.

From Hell, Hull and Halifax, May The Good Lord Deliver Us. The famous line originates in the Beggars' Litany, an old saying popular in the 17th century. The proverb had taken its origin "from the severe measures adopted by the magistrates of Hull and Halifax, at various times, to suppress vice".

It is best-known from a poem by John Taylor, who visited Hull in 1622 and wrote a description of the town in verse. However, it may already have been well known in Taylor's time. James Joseph Sheahan, in his history of Hull (1864), wrote: 'In it he (Taylor) alludes to the well-known line in the beggar and vagrants' litany – "From Hell, Hull, and Halifax, good Lord deliver us;" and also to the "Hull cheese ... the mightiest ale in England."'

Four hundred years ago, the Halifax Gibbet was among the most feared instruments of execution in the whole country. The machine looked and worked like a proto-guillotine, with an axe head mounted on a heavy wooden block, attached to an upright wooden frame. Petty criminals could find themselves strapped to the gibbet for stealing as little as 13-and-a-half pence. No wonder Halifax had such a frightening reputation.

Men do not wish deliverance from the town. The town's nam'd Kingston, Hull's the furious river, And from Hull's dangers I say Lord deliver. Why Hull was included in the litany is not so obvious. Most modern accounts suggest it was because of a notorious old gaol, but in Taylor's telling, the line is connected primarily to the river:

'Men do not wish deliverance from the town. The town's nam'd Kingston, Hull's the furious river, And from Hull's dangers I say Lord deliver.'

He may have had in mind an old tradition that in Hull, felons were tied to gibbets at low tide and left to drown as the river rose. Alternatively, the line may allude to the terror brought about by navy press gangs, which snatched young men from the town's streets and bars and pressed them into service onboard ships. In 1597, parliament passed the Vagabonds Act, which promoted press-ganging as a suitable punishment for vagrants. As Howard Peach writes in *Curious Tales of Old East Yorkshire*: 'Hull had its vagrants whipped and stocked, and some of its prisoners drowned on gibbets in the flood tide, or lost and tortured in the Tudor block house ... then came the press gang. There was plenty in Hull to promote anxiety.'

Taylor was known as the Water Poet because he spent much of his time as a boatman on the Thames. His poem is called 'Part of this Summer's Travels: Or News From Hell, Hull and Halifax'.

In a section called, A Very Merry-Wherry-Ferry
Voyage, he writes:

'There is a Proverb, and a Prayer withal,

That we may not to three strange places fall:

From Hull, from Halifax, from Hell, 'tis thus,

From all these three, Good Lord deliver us.

There is a Proverb, and a Prayer withal,

That we may not to three strange places fall:

From Hull, from Halifax, from Hell, 'tis thus,

From all these three, Good Lord deliver us.

This praying Proverb's meaning to set down,

Men do not wish deliverance from the Town,

The towns nam'd Kingston, Hull's the furious River:

And from Hull's dangers, I say Lord deliver.

At Halifax, the law so sharp doth deal,

That whoso more than 13 Pence doth steal,

They have a jyn that wondrous quick and well,

Sends thieves all headless unto Heav'n or Hell.

From Hell each man says, Lord deliver us.'

*   *   *

In Nov 2017 I attended the World Medical Association Conference on *End of Life Care* at The Vatican City in the shadow of St Peter's Square. Many countries in the world have been faced with crucial policy debates regarding euthanasia, physician assisted suicide and end of life issues especially in recent years. Increasing life expectancy, meteoric improvements in life-saving medical technology, internet revolution - all these have brought the issues to the forefront of global community. Medical advances like crypto-freezing even point towards the possibility of immortality. The conference actively explored and analysed the developments of policies surrounding these. The debates were led by medical professionals, legal authorities, palliative care experts, religious leaders, scholars and philosophers. Also, Pope Francis made a valuable contribution.

We had a wonderful tour of the Sistine Chapel, which is the traditional venue of the conclave to elect new popes, decorated by the illustrious frescoes of Michelangelo about the creation of the world and The Last Judgement. The gala dinner was held in the adjacent Vatican Museum, which is an important example of neoclassical architecture - the lavish gallery, monumental statues from the Roman period in the niches and an ornamental display of collection of sculptural portraits. The striking statue of Augustus, from the first century depicting the victorious emperor and the colossal effigy of the Nile stood out.

19

Court of Appeal Ruling - Justice Prevailed

Fiat justicia ruat caelum

(Let justice be done though the heavens fall)

The case of Dr Bawa-Garba shook the entire medical profession and the British Medical Association. In 2011, at Royal Leicester Infirmary, 6 year-old Jack Alcock tragically died of sepsis while under the treatment of the team including Dr Bawa-Garba. I express my deepest sympathy to the family in this regard. On the basis of the inquest, the CPS charged Dr BG and two nurses with gross negligence manslaughter. In 2015, BG and one of the nurses were convicted with BG receiving 2 year suspended sentence. Her appeal was refused.

In 2017, The Medical Practitioners Tribunal Service found BG's fitness to practice impaired and suspended her for a year. The GMC appealed this decision and in this January the high court upheld the appeal, erasing Dr BG from the medical register.

The concatenation of events, raised a myriad of complex questions. The key issues were - GMC's approach to appeal against MTPS judgement, absence of any consideration for the systemic failures admitted by the Trust, interpretation and application of gross negligence and manslaughter law in medical profession and use of personal reflective learning material against the doctor. The aftermath was that the profession lost its confidence in the regulator GMC. The impact of high court judgement was like the fallout of the Chernobyl nuclear accident. This could lead to practice of defensive medicine. Lord Denning's view is pertinent. 'We should be doing a disservice to the community at large if we were to impose liability on hospitals and doctors for everything that happens to go wrong. Doctors would be led to think more of their own safety than the good of the patients. Initiative would be stifled and confidence shaken… we must insist on due care for the patient at every point, but we must not condemn as negligence that which is only misadventure ([1957]1 WLR at 595 in Bolam v Friern Hospital Management Committee and in Roe v Minister of Health. In March 2018, Dr BG was given right of appeal and the BMA applied to assist the court. On 13 August, the court of appeal overturned the high court's decision, allowing BG to resume her career.

In 1998, GP Dr Narasinga Rao, while working at an Out of Hours Service in Wrexham admitted that his telephonic advice to the wife of a psychiatric patient was below standard. Later, the patient died of respiratory depression due to an accidental drug overdose. The GMC found him guilty of serious professional misconduct. On appeal, Rao v GMC [UKPC 65] (09 December 2002), the Privy Council ruled – 'There was undoubted negligence but something more was required to constitute serious professional misconduct and to attach the stigma of such a finding to a doctor of 25 years standing with a hitherto unblemished career.'

In the post-Shipman era, during Hyde-Six trial, the GMC attempted to use 'retrospectoscope' but failed. *Nullum crimen, nulla poena sine praevia lege poenali* (No ex post-facto laws).

Human Rights Act Article 6 – Right to Fair Trial

Everyone is entitled to a fair and public hearing within a reasonable time by an independent and impartial tribunal established by the law. With all the negative publicity preceding the high court trial, I doubt Dr Bawa-Garba did not get a fair trial. The trial was more of a televisual spectacle than an exercise of democratic justice. The doctor worked in very difficult and challenging conditions and made an error.

Article 11- *Everyone has the right, individually and in association with others, to the lawful exercise of his profession.* Although proportional reprimand is warranted for the doctor, to deprive her from practising for the rest of her life is like bringing back capital punishment. It is like banning from driving any driver involved in fatal accident, for the rest of his life.

Magna Carta Clause 40 guarantees impartial administration of justice. *Nulli vendemus, nulli negabimus aut differemus rectum aut justiciam* (to no one will we sell, to no one will we deny or delay right or justice). I think the GMC should not make the founding fathers King John and Archbishop Langton turn in their graves.

There has only been one doctor who was infallible - Pope John XXI (13th Century); all of us are bound to err. Whatever be the allegations against the doctor, passion should not give way to reason. In the 21st century, the star chamber of the medical profession should set an example to the rest of the world by upholding the Rule of Law and Human Rights.

*   *   *

Cremation

Cremation is a method of final disposition of a dead body through burning. Cremation may serve as a funeral or post-funeral rite and as an alternative to the burial or interment of an intact dead body. In some countries, including India and Nepal, cremation on an open-air pyre is an ancient tradition. In the post-Shipman era, cremation became a matter of paramount public and professional importance. Since the body will be burnt to ashes, the document is the last one of relating to that person.

Completing the cremation documentation has always been complex, complicated and time-consuming. I took great care in the process. In November 2014, the Medical Referee of The Crematorium, wrote to me:

'In my opinion, this Form 4 is **a model** of how Form 4 should be completed. You answered all the questions in a full and informative manner. It would make my job, which I have done for over 40 years, a lot easier if all doctors completed Form 4 as competently as you have done.'

*   *   *

Cottage Hospital - Halfway House

Many patients envisage cottage hospitals as transit lounges. The existence of these hospitals has been historically determined rather than planned. Ever since the inception of the NHS, many reports have supported the theme of GPs having access to hospital beds, in which they can care for some of the patients. The need for cottage hospitals is due to multiple factors. There has been a significant rise in the longevity of life with the resultant increase in geriatric ailments, many of them are chronic debilitating problems which per se do not warrant acute hospital care. In many instances, people are admitted to acute wards not necessarily due to clinical indications but due to a lack of carer, poor housing conditions and for safety reasons.

The concept of a 'hospital without walls' was generated in 1961 in New Zealand. The French followed suit by community agencies called 'hospitalisation *a domicile*'. In Peterborough hospital, the 'home scheme' was tried. All these aimed at bringing care to the sick in their own beds in the comfort of their home. The transition from acute hospital care to this setting could be eased by cottage hospitals.

First and foremost, there is a significant shortage of hospital beds. Especially in winter time, hundreds of patients are left on trolleys from 8 to 32 hours. The economic cost of maintaining patients in high technology hospitals is far more than the cost of care in low profile, patient-friendly cottage hospitals. Cost constraints in hospital care have always pressed for the quest of cost-effective alternatives. Problem of hospital-acquired infections are too familiar. There is an element of psychological trauma associated with acute hospital care.

Time and again, GPs have resisted vigorously the closure of cottage hospitals. In 1989, Dr Goodridge and 23 other GPs took Tunbridge Wells Health Authority to court against the closure of cottage hospitals and the high court ruled in their favour. In 1997, when North & East Devon Health Authority tried to close Lynton cottage hospital, Drs Frankish and Ferrar took them to court and won.

The theme of decentralising and bringing the much needed care closer to home is worth pursuing even though it is not panacea for all the medical needs of the community. Since home-based care is close to the heart of medical professionals and popular among the public, cottage hospitals ought to stay and act as halfway houses.

*　　　　　　　*　　　　　　　*

Private Way

Having worked in the NHS for over three decades, not even a week has passed without adverse report of costs in NHS care. The main source remains taxation although some readjustments from other departments are involved as well. Compared to European countries, the UK has the fewest hospital beds, except for Portugal. In 1998, the Chief Inspector of Prisons remarked that the public sector prisons could learn many lessons from prisons run on contract by private firms. Similar initiatives involving private contractors are worth trying with hospitals. In Australia, impressive results have been achieved with hospitals that are publicly funded but privately operated.

20

Locum Doctor

'To get away from one's working environment is, in a sense, to get away from one's self; and this is often the chief advantage of travel and change.'

Charles Horton Cooley

In the good old days, working as a locum doctor was almost similar to working on the Trans-Siberian Railway under the Stalin regime. In his book *New Kind of Doctor,* Dr Julian Tudor Hart described his experience in South Wales: 'Acting as a locum in Ferndale, Rhondda, in 1960, I saw about 60 patients in the morning session, another 60 in the evening, and visited 25 patients at home.' The locum landscape has changed a lot since then.

When I was in full-time practice running my own surgery, I used to hold a practice meeting before I went on holiday. I insisted that all staff must look after the locum doctor better than me since he was not familiar to the practice and area. Also, I used to ring from abroad in between to check his welfare.

After helping out colleagues as a locum doctor for many years, I noticed various shortcomings and irregularities. I also have discussed these with my locum colleagues and would highlight the problems which locum doctors face. A locum does not have the luxury of an existing knowledge and relationship with the patient, cannot do any follow up of the patient once he finishes the clinic. He has to ensure that he covers all eventualities in that short space of time. But the regular GP has all the advantages of starting the race in pole position.

I am citing examples:

On arrival at a practice, a locum found the practice team was in a meeting. The receptionist asked the doctor to hold on in the waiting room full of patients. After a few minutes, the doctor approached the receptionist whether he could go into the consulting room just to escape from the waiting room. The reply was blunt, "I have no authority; you will have to wait here until the manager is free." If it was a workman on a call out, he would have left long back and sent a bill for wasting his time. Another doctor, on arrival, was welcomed by the practice manager and taken to the consulting room. After two minutes banal exchange of formalities, he handed over 'Locum Folder' which was as thick as Yellow Pages and left saying 'All the information is here' without even showing him where the toilet was. A doctor was doing locum for one week; during tea break, he joined other members of the practice team. They were all chatting away without even recognising his very existence. Feeling like a pariah, he made a silent exit. A doctor passed belittling comments to staff – "Dr A is too slow, Dr B is prescribing too much antibiotics" etc.

In many practices, the receptionist answers phone calls with, "Dr Jones is on holidays. I can give you an appointment with the locum." Even the doctor's name is not mentioned. Patients get the impression that they are seeing a stand-in second grade doctor. This increases the risk of dissatisfaction and complaints. Many practices simply put 'Locum Doctor' (no name) on the board. Many GPs comment like, "I was away; it was only a locum who dealt with that" which sows seeds of doubt in patient's minds.

Often, the locum doctor works away out of his town. He does not know the practice, local arrangements and hospitals, the area, social situation etc. Quite often the host practice makes a 'mountain out of a molehill' about the trivial pitfalls of locum and a whispering campaign follows. Just to cite some instances - the locum doctor parked in the slot of doctors' car park. He was asked to move his car and park elsewhere, even though he was covering a doctor in that practice. When a locum went in, many family photos and cards of the incumbent doctor were displayed on the crowded table. The locum slightly moved them around to make adequate room for examination. After the clinic, the regular doctor raised an issue against the locum. When I used to employ a locum, I used to clear my desk to ensure that the locum works with a clean slate. The toilet was a bit dirty; locum overheard a staff saying, "It must be the locum." A group practice booked a locum for 4 hours, but surgery finished 30 minutes prior; the locum stayed in his room for the contacted 4 hours; the practice would pay only for 3.5 hours; the tug of war went on for weeks. The locum had to threaten with small claims court proceeding and only then got paid in full. They wouldn't dare to try it on a plumber. Some practices take ages to pay locums although the locum invoiced them for payment within 7 days. The list goes on…

Many of the instances cited can land the Practice on the wrong side of the law and ethics. The Declaration of Geneva states, 'My colleagues will be my brothers and sisters'. It is essential that the regular GPs give prior instruction to staff to treat locums like themselves. The International Code of Medical Ethics spells out, 'A physician shall behave to his colleagues as he would have them behave towards him'. Health and Safety at Work Act (1974) imposes a general duty on employers to ensure, as far as reasonably practicable the health, safety and welfare of all employees. This applies to human behaviour and physical environment. The regular GPs need to treat their professional brothers with care, compassion and consideration. Locum doctors trying to earn their daily bread should be treated with dignity and respect.

The bright side is there were some exemplary Practices. Prime examples were Beverley & Molescroft Surgery and Central Surgery, Barton, where I have helped out over many years. The doctors, manager and all staff made me feel welcome. They treated me as part of the team, valued my input and opinion and above all treated me with dignity and respect. Henry Ford remarked, 'If everyone is moving forward together, then success takes care of itself'. The end result was I always put in 110% endeavour at these practices.

*   *   *

2006

My daughter, Rowena, got admission to the School of Medicine, St Andrews, Fife, Scotland. It is oldest medical school in Scotland, founded in 1412. The medical school teaches pre-clinical medicine with students completing clinical teaching at different medical schools in the UK.

St Andrews has quite a history for such a small place. Legend claims that the town was so called because it harboured the relics of St Andrew, which were brought here by a bishop, St Rule, from Patras in Achaea. It is the birthplace of_golf, and the Royal and Ancient Club, which was created in 1754, has been the headquarters of golf ever since. The Duke and Duchess of Cambridge were the recent famous alumni of St Andrews. The College Chapel contains the pulpit where John Knox preached, and in the grounds there is a thorn tree reputedly planted by Mary, Queen of Scots.

In the early sixteenth century the castle was the home of Cardinal David Beaton, the Catholic martyr, or the bloody oppressor of Protestantism, according to one's viewpoint. He was a very important man and became Mary Queen of Scots' chancellor after she was crowned. In the early days of the Reformation, Beaton was ruthless in stamping-out the slightest hint of Lutheran heresy, and in the process created the earliest Protestant martyrs in Scotland. Below St Andrews Castle is a 'bottle shaped' dungeon. This is where Cardinal Beaton imprisoned Protestants, and when they went mad in the darkness and screamed for help, he had them hanged.

I used to make regular trips to visit Rowena on weekends. I stayed in a nearby B&B, run by Len and Marjorie who were in their late sixties. On evenings when I returned, Len would bring a nightcap - his favourite Oban whisky - and narrate various folktales of his life. Oban is single malt 43% *ABV*. The nose offers soft smoke, heather honey, toffee and a whiff of seashore. Spicy, cooked fruits on the palate, with malt, oak and a little smoke. The finish is rounded and aromatic, with spices and oak. Occasionally, Marjorie also joined in. One day, she showed me something she got her from her grandmother who worked with Queen Victoria. It was the Christmas lunch menu of Her Majesty, at Windsor castle, 1899:

Negus

Potages

Consomme' a' la Monaco

Potage Du Berry

Poissons

Filets de Sile a' la Vassant

Esperlans frits, sauce Verneuil

Entre'e

Cotelettes de Volaille a' laYork

Relebe's

Dinde a' la Chipolata

Roast Beef

Chine of Pork

Entreeme'ts

Asperges sauce Hollandaise

Plum Pudding, German Custard

Mince Pies

Gele'e d'Orange a' l'Anglaise

Malt whisky

Just 12 courses only; Queen Victoria's menu was influenced by influx of French chefs in 1840. Even at the ripe old age of 79, she tucked in, got indigestion as usual and had a nap after the meal.

    *   *   *

Dr Wolverson – scapegoat of the system?

The *Daily Mail*, May 25, 2019, pages 30-31 carried the story of Dr Wolverson, a locum GP being out of work after receiving a letter from GMC that he was being investigated for racial discrimination and could result in being struck off, following a complaint regarding consultation one year back, where he requested a Muslim woman to lift her veil to get a clear history when she brought her 5 year-old daughter. The woman obliged his request but later her husband made a complaint.

He said, "Unfortunately I am a locum GP and no one will employ you while you are under investigation by the GMC." After 23 years of unblemished career, he is on the precipice of his medicinal life. Although capital punishment was abolished by the parliament, GMC has its own version of the professional annihilation of doctors. All the while, the country has a shortage of 6000 GPs. *That* rings alarm bells across the profession.

The GMC's kneejerk reaction raises fundamental questions:

(a) **Presumption of innocence** - In the Anglo-Saxon legal set up 'All are innocent until proven otherwise'. This is a fundamental tenet of British democratic edifice and keystone of the arch of civilized society.

(b) **Legal equality**- All individuals have the same rights before the law. In this instance, the complainant is given anonymity while the defendant is subjected to wide publicity with his photographs in national papers, which will adversely affect his career whatever the outcome is.

(c) **Article 6 of the Human Rights Act** – *Everyone is entitled to a fair and public hearing within a reasonable time by an independent and impartial tribunal established by the law.* If Dr Wolverson's name is tagged, it is tantamount to presuming guilt before trial and verdict. This is putting prejudice before justice.

(d) **Article 11 of the Human Rights Act** - *Everyone has the right, individually and in association with others, to the lawful exercise of his profession.* The prospective employers are not offering him jobs; this deprives him of his right to practice his profession. Human rights are integral to the daily life of every person on this planet and depriving them, is like suffocation. Doctors also should be treated with dignity and respect and their human rights ought to be respected. **Estoppel -** *Legal principle that bars a party from denying or alleging a certain fact owing to that party's previous conduct, allegation or denial.* The rationale is to prevent injustice owing to inconsistency or fraud. Once the patient (in this case the parent) agrees, the scenario is legally bound by estoppel. Estoppel forms part of the rules of equity originally administered in Chancery courts. **Magna Carta Libertatum (1215) - Clause 39 -** *No free man ... will be deprived of his standing in any way.... except by the lawful judgement of his equals or by the law of the land.* **Clause 40 -** *To no one will we sell, to no one deny or delay right or justice.* Dr Wolverson was deprived of his standing and his right to justice was delayed. The GMC should not cause King John and the Archbishop of Canterbury, Steven Langton, to turn in their graves; let them sleep comfortably in peace. **GMC Consent: patients and doctors working together (2 June 2008)** – Para 7- *You should tailor your approach to discussion according to (a) their needs, wishes and priorities (b) their level of knowledge about, and understanding of their condition, prognosis and treatment options (c) the nature of the condition (d) the complexity of treatment (e) the nature and level of risk associated with the investigation/treatment.* Para 10 - *You should explore matters with patients, listen to their concerns... encourage them to ask questions.* Para 32 - *You should do your best to understand the patient's views and preferences, adverse outcomes..... You should discuss these issues.*

As per the newspaper report, the doctor was endeavouring to put these in practice by attempting to get a clear history and sound clinical assessment. **Best interest -** The doctor has acted in the <u>best interest</u> of the patient (child). He has been thorough and made a conscientious effort to take good history rather than a cursory examination.

In 2006, the Home Secretary, Jack Straw, requested Muslim women to lift veils in his weekly surgery in Blackburn in 'face-to-face' meetings.

In Sept 2013, Judge Peter Murphy at Blackfriars Crown Court ruled that a Muslim woman had to remove her veil to give evidence. In these instances, the fundamental issue was to seek effective communication. While this issue was raised in different platforms, instead of sleep-walking, the GMC ought to have taken pro-active steps with anticipation and foresight since in some areas the population has significantly high ethnic minorities. This is of paramount importance. The 'social norms' cannot simply be 'cut and pasted' into a courtroom, airport security and especially medical consultations where nearly one third of all consultations would involve the examination of bare body parts or orifices.

Current GMC guidance is loose jargon. In a 10 minute consultation, there is little time for exploring religious beliefs. Even if somebody does, it may be misconstrued or misinterpreted. Moreover there are various religions and subsects - Hindus, Sikhs, Buddhists etc. The vast majority of Muslims I have come across in 27 years of general practice, are British in thought, word and deed and have British values and exhibit mutual respect. In the absence of clear-cut policy, to incriminate Dr Wolverson, was witch-hunting.

We must not look at 1947 incident with 1954 spectacles.

Denning LJ, **Roe** v **Minister of Health** *[1954]*

2 AII ER 131

This decision by *Court of Appeal* has significant impact throughout common law. It was also worth noting Dr Amra Bone, Britain's only female sharia court judge's view that covering one's face is not obligatory for Muslim women.

William Osler, one of the *great* physicians of the past, remarked, 'Listen to your patient; he is telling you the diagnosis.' In **Glass v UK** [2004] EHRR 341 and **Tysiac v Poland** [2007] EHRR 947, the duty to involve patients in decisions relating to their treatment have been well recognized in the judgements. Dr Wolverson was trying his best to do so. In a busy walk-in-centre, working as a solo GP, with constraint of time, under duress of circumstances, Dr Wolverson has acted reasonably and proportionately. He will pass the **Custom Test** as in **Hunter v Hanley** [1955] S.C. 200.

In order to establish liability in circumstances where deviation from normal practice is alleged, three facts have to be established.

(a) It must be proved that there is a usual and normal practice.

(b) It must be proved that the defender has not adopted that practice.

(c) It must be established that the course the professional has adopted is one which no professional person of ordinary skill would have taken if he/she had been acting with ordinary care. Most of the GPs would have acted similarly in the given circumstances. It is fairly clear that the doctor acted in good faith to give the best possible care. The lack of *mens rea* (the intention or knowledge of any wrongdoing) is explicit. This doctor would also pass the **Bolam Test** as in ***Bolam v Friern Hospital Management Committee*** [1957] 2 AII ER 118.

The scenario is not about race, religion or culture. This is an affront on a GP by a disgruntled relative. The chain of events of this cancer eroding medical practice (patient complaint > unreasonable delay > doctor's loss of livelihood and damage of reputation/career > GMC hearing > no adverse outcome in most cases) must be severed. Whatever the allegations be against the doctor, passion should not give way to reason. Proportionality, common sense and reasonableness must prevail. In the 21st century, the star chamber of the profession should set an example to the rest of the world by fair trial and upholding the Rule of Law and Human Rights.

*   *   *

Chaperone

One of the ongoing problems in general practice is the presence of chaperones at consultations. So many complaints, premature termination of careers, breakdown of family relationships and suicides have happened surrounding this issue. For any doctor, an accusation of inappropriate behaviour towards a patient is devastating and the consequences can be far reaching. Cases can take many months, and often years, to resolve, by which time the doctor concerned may have been through criminal, civil, and General Medical Council (GMC) proceedings as well as facing adverse publicity in the media.

The Ayling report, published September 2004, (about chaperoning) found a lack of common understanding of the purpose and use of chaperones across the NHS. It recognized that chaperones were used in various settings and circumstances with differing levels of risk to patients and healthcare professionals. It recommended that:

(a) Trained chaperones should be available to all patients having intimate examinations. Untrained administrative staff or family or friends of the patient should not be expected to act as chaperones.

(b) The presence of a chaperone must be the patient's choice and they must be able to decline a chaperone if they wish.

(c) All NHS trusts need to set out a clear chaperone policy and should ensure that patients are aware of it and that it is adequately funded. The report recognized that for primary care a policy will have to take into account issues such as one to one consultations in patients' homes and the capacity of practices to meet the requirements of an agreed policy.

The Medical Defence Union went one step further, advising that doctors should try to use chaperone for eye examinations. The recommendations in this report raised more questions than answers, without addressing the fundamental issues. They are loose and lukewarm and look good on paper in an ideal world which is Utopia. *The Oxford English Dictionary* defines a chaperone as 'a person, especially on older woman, who ensures propriety by accompanying a young unmarried woman on social occasions'. My view is this was a definition suiting the Victorians. Now most young women want full freedom and independence to go out. The society has changed dramatically.

What is routine in one place can be alien in another. There are cultural and religious differences to consider. For example, some women want their abdomen palpated over clothing. During GP consultations, nurses may be busy doing blood tests or cervical smears etc. Also, in many small surgeries, the nurse's availability is limited.

Do we ask every patient who walks through the door to have a chaperone? If we ask one patient and do not ask the next one, that itself can be construed as differential treatment and discriminatory. Consultation is a two-way process; both patients and doctors have rights. As doctors, we have to follow universally accepted norms and practices. Health professionals need to stick to a policy of using a chaperone if they feel it necessary for whatsoever reasons. The General Medical Council Advice on Intimate Examinations (2001) said doctors can invite a relative or friend to be present (contradictory in Ayling report). Are we supposed to take a chaperone on a home visit? Where do we get one? What do we do if an elderly confused lady living on her own needs urgent intimate examination or suppository?

Many disputes arise from the interpretation of consent. In most instances, doctors try their best to explain what they intend to do during the process of consultation. The legal principle, 'When the patient gives no specific instructions, the rule applied in English Law is that [consent is given] once the patient is informed in broad terms of the nature of the intended procedure and validates the consent' – **Chatterton *v* Gerson** [1981] 1 ALL ER 257-65.

With the Covid-19 crisis, most consultations are in a remote setting with a few video consultations. Most firms now use audio/video to 'improve quality and prevent fraud'. Many street crimes are solved on the evidence from CCTVs. It would be in the interest of all parties that consultations also are videoed or audioed in future. After all, we live in the 21st century.

21

(2016) Hail Shakespeare - Mythical, Magical, Medicinal Wizard

'Every household in the English speaking world is not properly furnished unless it contains a copy of the Holy Bible or the work of Shakespeare.'

Harrison

My fascination with Shakespeare is lifelong. I read *The Complete Works of Shakespeare* by age 12. I had acted in his plays enacted at my college. When my articles got published, a friend of mine used to e-mail me. 'Well done, Thomas Shakespeare'.

While the world was paying homage to Shakespeare on his 400th death anniversary, it was poignant to ponder over his everlasting contributions to the field of medicine. He was not just an English playwright but a global citizen and phenomenon. He is revered across the world; his plays have been translated into 180 languages. References to physicians, diseases and treatments occur in most of his plays. Although he had no formal medical training, taking into consideration his medical knowledge, we should put him on the same pedestal as the great physicians like Hippocrates and Galen.

In the early 16th century, when Shakespeare lived in London, the city was overcrowded and unsanitary. The streets were littered with garbage, rodents ruled the roads and death dominated daily life. Hygiene was such a rare quality that even the queen only bathed once a month. Against the backdrop of all this phantasmagoria of horrible nonsense, he wrote his plays. His unfathomable in-depth understanding of the dysfunctions of the body and mind were deliciously depicted in his works. Shakespeare gained medical knowledge on his own since he wrote most of his plays even before his eldest daughter Susanne got married to Joseph Hall, a physician, in 1607.

He described the ailments affecting all systems of the body and mind. Even after four centuries, his works are beacons of eternal learning across the globe. I shall give a glimpse of his vision:

Psychosis -

> *In this the dagger which I see before me,*
>
> *A dagger of the mind, a false creation.*
>
> *Macbeth, II, I, 38*

Old age -

> *A good leg will fall; a straight back will droop;*
>
> *A fair face will wither; a full eye will wax hollow.*
>
> *King Henry V, V, ii, 155*

Burnout due to excessive workload -

> *Long sitting to determine poor men's causes*
>
> *Hath made me full of sickness and disease.*
>
> *King Henry IV, IV, vii, 82*

Care Homes -

> *We will bestow you in some better place,*
>
> *Fitter for sickness and for crazy age.*
>
> *King Henry VI, III, II, 88*

Rabies -

> *... take heed of yonder dog!*
>
> *Look when he fawns, he bites;*
>
> *His venom tooth will rankle to the death.*
>
> *King Richard III, I, ii, 289*

Epilepsy -

And when the fit was on him I did mark

How he did shake.

Julius Caesar, I, II, 120

There are picturesque descriptions of Caesarean section in *Macbeth*, pregnancy symptoms in *Love's Labour's Lost* and plague in *Troilus and Cressida*. The list is so vast, elaborate and laborious.

In an era when there was no electricity, computing and revelatory technology, this man-wonder created his works in immaculate style, crystal-clear clarity and precision with supreme aplomb. Not a day passes without reference to Shakespeare - stories being told, plays being enacted, works being read, research into his works, people visiting his house and so on. The hero lives on, in the hearts and minds of billions across the globe.

Shakespeare has been the best honourable 'medical knowhow' ever, who brilliantly enlightened the world of the ailments and maladies in dramatically adventurous, linguistically gorgeous style. As a genius who analysed the cliffs and cavers of the brain, tides and currents of the heart and translated those into galaxy of plays, his place is unique. We all need to salute and shout out from rooftops 'Hail Shakespeare, mythical, magical, medicinal wizard'.

*   *   *

2016 - Passing on the Baton

In April 2016, my daughter Rowena took the MRCGP (Member of the Royal College of General Practitioners) at the ceremony at the RCGP headquarters in London. It was a proud privilege to take part in the ceremony with my wife Mary, son Thomas and Rowena's partner, Dr James (Senior Registrar in Urology).

The Royal College has 50,000 members worldwide. The college is committed to high standard learning tools and developing educational standards in specialty training. Ongoing research is at the forefront of the college. There are various activities undertaken by the college – improving overall experience of patients, lobbying the government and helping to shape health policy.

She has entered the arena marked by a plethora of contrasting and complex challenges than when I entered general practice. Patient expectations and demands have rocketed. The profession is under multi-pronged attack from the press, politicians and the public. The internet revolution has made many patients feel that they know best. There seems to be a generalised lack of respect towards the profession. The trans-Atlantic wave of litigation is spreading fast here also. A third of the GPs are due to retire in 5 years. Too many shepherds are controlling the herd from various angles - GMC, CCG, NICE, CQC etc.

Albert Einstein remarked, 'It has become appallingly obvious that our technology has exceeded our humanity.' It is true about general practice also. With the advent of modern technology appointments are better organised, investigations better and quicker and we have remarkable improvements in cancer care. Professional development opportunities are a lot better than in my early days. Annual appraisal is more methodical. Under the 'GP Forward View', the government pledged £206 million to tackle 5000 GP recruitment target and an increase in GP funding of £2.4 billion per year by 2020/21.

Passing the baton to next generation is a productive, protracted and painstaking phenomenon. When you run the relay and pass on the baton, there is a sense of optimism that the person running the next stage of the race can run faster and longer. I was pleased for her to join me into the vocation. I have loosened the grip on the baton and let her hold on to it but not given away completely yet.

22

(2017) UK City of Culture

'Culture opens the sense of beauty.'

Ralph Waldo Emerson

After living in Hull for quarter of a century, I was pleased to take part in the celebrations. The City of Culture was active throughout 2017 and lasts till the end of 2020. The theme was 'A city coming out of the shadows'.

Season 1 (January-March) *Made in Hull*. On 1 January 2017, the celebration started with a fireworks display at Humber Estuary. The BBC reported that in the first week, 342,000 took part in the opening events. Multimedia and light projections were put onto Victoria square and landmark buildings. Season 2 (April-June) *Roots & Routes*. This was an emphasis on Hull as a gateway, celebrating migration and flux. Season 3 (July-September) *Freedom*. Recognition of the role of Hull's famous son William Wilberforce, who started the movement to abolish slave trade and combatting abuse of human rights. At the Freedom Festival, a musical extravaganza, former United

Nations Secretary-General Kofi Annan (2001 Nobel Prize winner for Peace), gave the Wilberforce lecture and awarded the Wilberforce Medallion. Season 4 (October-December) *Tell the world*. The Turner Prize ceremony was held in December 2017. The emphasis was for redefining the city for the future.

*   *   *

2017 marked the most memorable event in our family. On 6th August, Rowena and James got married at Our Lady & St Herbert Church, Windermere. At the bride's father's speech, I surprised the couple and the audience with a gift from the Eternal City of Rome - The Highest among the high priests of all, the Supreme Pontiff of the Universal Catholic Church, His Holiness Pope Francis's Apostolic Blessing 'that the marriage consecrated at the altar will be blessed each day with divine graces'. Shortly after, James was promoted as Consultant Urologist as well.

*   *   *

2018 - In November 2018, The Royal College of General Practitioners, Humber & Ridings Faculty shortlisted me for the *Outstanding Contribution to General*

Practice Award, but I narrowly missed out on the accolade.

23

Renting Nightmare

'Res ipsa loquitur.'
Cicero
(The thing speaks for itself.)

On 1st September 2017, since our house was being refurbished, we rented a flat from the letting agent Beercocks Letting Agents, Hull.

After occupying, there were several ongoing problems with the failure of hot water, central heating, water leak etc. After reporting these problems, the response was very poor. I had to complain to the East Riding of Yorkshire Council to get things sorted out.

We were due to vacate on 30 November 2018. The chain of contacts are outlined as follows:

22/11/2018 - my e-mail - I am available at 11.30am on 30/11/18 to hand over keys and metre readings etc.

22/11/2018 - reply - keys to be dropped off at one of our offices; within couple of days will carry out final inspection.

30/11/2018 - I handed over the keys to Hessle office.

11/12/2018 - my email - 11 days since vacating; can you send deposit.

11/12/2018 - reply - will speak to colleague who does the inspection.

20/12/2018 - email - completed checkout, contacted landlord and awaiting response.

02/01/2019 - my email - more than a month since vacated; not received deposit; can you refund without delay.

17/01/2019 - reply - tried to meet up with landlord; waited 20 minutes at property for her, not available over phone; e-mailed her; she feels property needs some additional cleaning.

18/01/2019 - my email - Property 100 years old, ongoing significant deficiencies, engaged cleaners to clean and tidy landlord not seen the property prior to purchase, any issue ought to have been brought to my attention at time of vacating, not after weeks and months; not refunding deposit unreasonable and unacceptable.

18/01/2019 - reply to Branch Manager - my email forwarded, landlord not responding and not replying; flat needs some additional cleaning, maybe we could return all except £300.

20/01/2019 - e-mail to me - awaiting response from Manager.

29/01/2109 - my e-mail - deeply disappointed, landlord's actions irresponsible, inconsiderate and insensitive… withholding deposit causing financial distress, emotional injury and obstruction of HMRC payment. Request full settlement by 30/01/2019.

30/01/2019 – reply - met with landlord at property, needs some cleaning; can you send receipt of cleaning.

I scanned and sent cleaning bill of £256.

01/02/2019 - reply: landlord thinks property needs additional cleaning.. would like cleaners to re-attend…

05/02/2019 - my e-mail - was waiting to discuss with the cleaners who did the job. If this information was passed on promptly on vacating, I could have got them without delay; can you send photos and quote?

28/02/2019 – reply - after speaking to landlord, list of costs £1350.

05/03/2019 - in response to your e-mail, I wish to submit the following:

My reference to 'you' means the firm Beercocks.

The demands mentioned in your e-mail are unreasonable, unjustifiable and untimely. Regarding the bulbs - for prudent and judicious use of energy, the fused bulbs were not replaced. However, due to the fact that the washing machine was faulty, the laundry bills have far exceeded £30. Also, I had to replace the letter box since the lock was faulty.

The wardrobe was forgotten by accident since it was in the box room. You were well aware that belonged to me. By civic responsibility and common law any reasonable person would have displayed the onus and obligation to alert the owner promptly rather than destroying somebody else's property. I cannot comment on any other matters cited, since I handed over the keys 3 months back and personnel have been in the property day and night.

Although on 22 Nov 18, I e-mailed you to meet at the property on 30 Nov 18 (day of vacating) to hand over the keys, the response was 'to drop the keys in any of the offices and within a couple of days of receiving them we will carry out the final inspection'. I duly handed over the keys at 1530 on 30 Nov 18 to Hessle office. I had looked after the property like my own home and ensured it was left in the best possible state on leaving.

I would have liked to hand over the keys in person to you at the property. But I obliged your request trusting the promise of final inspection within two days. If the inspection was going to be any longer, I would have acted differently. You <u>deprived me</u> <u>deliberately of my basic right to verify the state of affairs on vacating.</u> This was **gross breach of trust.**

You ought to have returned the deposit within 10 days of vacating. Although I sent further e-mails, I was given various excuses. On 1/2/19 you sent e-mail regarding cleaning and I sent you the cleaning bill. Your latest e-mail is self- contradictory.

I also wish to remind you that, to start with you were discriminatory in the fact that you put much higher deposit than the usual (you acknowledged that in your e-mail 18/01/19). Our tenancy was marred by a catalogue of problems involving failure of central heating, hot water, washing machine etc making the stay miserable. There was a water leak near the main electricity switches causing considerable damage and destroying some of my important files. Although I reported, no action was taken. When the heating broke down, mushrooms started growing over the carpet in some areas. Only after reporting to East Riding Council, matters were temporarily but partially resolved.

In short: You have **breached Consumer Rights Act [2015]** by (a) *acting without due care and skill* – negligence (b) *taking unreasonable amount of time* of over three months to refund the deposit which was due in 10 days and still not done. **Unfair and dishonest trading behaviour** (as cited above in making me drop off the keys on false promise). I have been deceived.

The deposit was paid into your account from my Account No:....., Sort Code: ....I had waited for more than 3 months after vacating for the return of the deposit. Can you ensure the deposit is paid back into my account within 5 days? If this is not done, I will report all the irregularities during tenancy and after vacating to the Trading Standards. Also, I may be forced to take necessary steps to act in public interest so that potential tenants would not be subjected to similar unacceptable behaviour which do not suit a civilised society.

05/03/2019 – reply - claim now lodged with DPS

When I wrote to the Deposit Protection Scheme, they replied that they had released the deposit of £2250 back to letting agent.

So, after all these 'pillar to post' dealings, I still have not received the deposit back. I am bringing it to the attention of the public since this is a matter of public interest especially those planning to rent property.

The inordinate delays, delaying tactics by ever-changing goal posts and blatant disregard for set norms and practices, have resulted in financial loss and significant emotional distress. Justice has still been denied. I do not wish anybody to go through a similar nightmare.

24

Role Model

'Being a role model is about being true to myself.'

Idina Menzel

In March 2019, the world renowned *British Medical Journal* published an article which cited me as a role model; the first of its kind for any Hull doctor.

Thomas is articulate, brave and prepared to challenge authority. His articles are eloquent, passionate and often challenge conventional thinking in medicine. He has chaired educational meetings, taught medical students and provided support and inspiration for colleagues, particularly those facing criticism or burnout.

He is courteous and clever, yet always respectful of staff and patients, whom he treats as his equals. He examines patients with care and respect. Thomas has suffered some significant personal tragedies in his life, and yet he has managed to retain his dignity, values and sense of humour.

*   *   *

April 2019 - How a snail in the bottle came to define GPs' duty of care.

It is fascinating to recall that the modern law of negligence evolved following a trivial incident of consuming a fizzy drink in 1928 in Paisley, near Glasgow. I made a pilgrimage to the site of origin in November 2019. *Donoghue* v *Stevenson* [1932] AC 562, also known as the 'Snail in the bottle case' is one of the most celebrated and landmark cases in the British legal history. In 1928, Ms Amy Donoghue was invited by a friend to Well Meadow Café, Paisley. The friend bought her a ginger beer. Halfway through, Ms Donoghue felt something drastically wrong - a decomposed snail was in the beer. She later fell ill and developed gastroenteritis.

Donoghue sued the manufacturer, David Stevenson, in Court of Sessions, Scotland. The court dismissed the case due to lack of precedent and said there was no case to answer. She was granted leave to appeal. She went to the House of Lords, who passed the judgement in Donoghue's favour. The judgement established several legal principles:

The **'Neighbourhood Principle'** - Donoghue had received the drink as a gift; she was a 'neighbour' rather than a party to the contract.

'The rule that you are to love your neighbour becomes in law, you must not injure your neighbour... You must take reasonable care to avoid acts or omissions which you can reasonably foresee would be likely to injure your neighbour.

Who, then, in law is my neighbour? Persons who are so closely and directly affected by my act that I ought reasonably to have them in contemplation as being so affected when I am directing my mind to the acts or omissions which are called in question.'

- Lord Atkin

Duty of care - The case proved that the manufacturer has a duty of care to the consumers who use the products. Lord Atkin made it clear in *ratio decendi- a manufacturer of products which he sells…to reach the ultimate consumer in the form in which they left him… owes a duty to the consumer, to take reasonable care'*. This principle has later been applied in many laws including Trade Practice Act (Commonwealth, 1974). This is paramount importance in medical practice where thousands of drugs, equipment and vaccines are used on a daily basis.

Negligence - the House of Lords ruling confirmed that negligence is a tort. A plaintiff can take legal action against a respondent if the respondent's negligence causes injury or loss or damage to property.

Duty of care is a legal obligation imposed on an individual requiring that they adhere to a standard of reasonable care while performing any acts that could foreseeably harm others. It may be considered a formalisation of the social contract. The seminal English case that first introduced the concept of 'reasonable person' was *Vaughan* v *Menlove* [1837] 132

ER 490. Menlove built a haystack in his own land but near the boundary of Vaughan's cottage, in spite of being warned that it might catch fire. The hay caught fire and damaged the cottage. The Court ruled in Vaughan's favour – *We ought to rather adhere to the rule which requires in all cases a regard to caution such as a man of ordinary prudence would observe.*

Translating these into medical practice, all health professionals have a duty of care to themselves, patients, colleagues and 'neighbours' (those who are likely to come into contact during daily practice). This is applicable to every aspect of the work. In practice, always act in the best interest of patients, avoid act or omission which are likely to cause harm. Always put safety first - act within own competence. In reality, this composes of many issues - keeping knowledge and skills up to date, provide service at the standard of the reasonable person, use discretion to ensure that the service can be delivered safely, delegate work only when it is safe to do so, keep records accurate, protect confidentiality etc.

The duty of care is a standard in the law of negligence. It is a duty to act in the way a responsible person should act in the given circumstance and deviation from this could result in negligence. The duty of care can be owed by the individual or the establishment. The failure to use reasonable care can result in negligence.

In a nutshell, a young Scottish lady confronted the establishment and challenged the legal system with courage, conviction and confidence, achieving victory for herself and thereby establishing one of the key fundamental legal principles. This has been followed not only in the UK but also across most of the commonwealth, so almost two-thirds of the world. The statute of Amy Donoghue is placed across the road opposite Lord Atkin's judgement, in Paisley. Let us pay tribute to the brave lady Ms Amy Donoghue for being the catalyst to establish the norms of duty of care globally.

*   *   *

One of my medical schoolmates and close friend, Dr Mohan Tharakan, died in 2019. He was a dedicated and popular GP in Shiremoor. I used to cover his practice as locum on a number of occasions in the past. During those times, he would ring me and enquire about my well-being and ask me about certain patients he was worried about. He could not offload medical practice from his mind wherever he was. After a long career, he retired and spent six months in the UK and six months in India. In modern times, when courtesy and respect are in short supply, he was the very embodiment of both. His radiant smile and immaculate manners generated a positive flow of energy to those who came across him. Although he became a man by age, by choice he became a gentleman. Tennis was his craze. While in India, one day when he went to play tennis, he had a fall, sustained a head injury and died in hospital. MOHAN [**M**eticulous**, O**utpouring, **H**armonic, **A**ffectionate, **N**oble]. I cherish our long-term friendship and fellowship. *Requiesat in pace.*

'His life was gentle, and the elements so mixed in him, that nature might stand up and say to all the world "This was a man".'

Shakespeare (Julius Caesar)

25

2020 Vision - Revisited

'We do not learn; and what we call learning is only a process of recollection.'

Plato

My article in 1995, **GP's Central Role in Shaping Things to Come - 2020 Vision,** was runner-up in a national competition. After quarter of a century, I have travelled down memory lane to revisit this piece.

Ageing: 1995 - The increasing number of old people will prove to be a burden because more resources from society have to be diverted to cater for their needs. Ageism will be regarded as an offence. *Daily Mail,* **February 12, 2020** carries front page article - **New Chief Medical Officer warns of surge in elderly population**; reveals rural areas are struggling to cope; insists only a health revolution can avert emergency.

Home visits: 1995 - Traditional style home visits will cease. Visits will be limited to institutionalised patients. Also, ambulance doctors will do the visits, fully supported with other health professions. Now, the overwhelming mood among GPs is to abolish home visits. Also, many practices employ First Care Practitioners to do the home visits.

Loss of freedom: 1995 - Personal freedom will be increasingly under threat. Professional freedom will be curtailed by more and more codes of conduct. A myriad of newer rules and regulations have appeared like mushrooms affecting freedom and producing claustrophobic accountability.

Cost: Doctors will have to be more aware of cost factors. Choice of available resources will be the important parameter since resources are finite. Now, when we prescribe, if we get the 'cost warning', most try to prescribe suitable alternative. Also 'lumps and lumps' are dealt with additional funding route. Cost awareness is at the forefront of most dealings. The primary care network DES specifications stipulate that any extra funding has significant strings attached.

Alternative medicine: 1995 - Alternative medicine will continue to grow and will act as an opiate for those disillusioned with the orthodox kind. Alternative medicine is now widely used in many cases.

Computers: 1995 - Almost all practices will be computerised. There is no need to emphasize that all practices are now computerised.

1995 - The hardships and hazards of general practice will continue to rise, including violence and litigation. And so they are.

1995 - Psycho-somatic illnesses, the doctor-patient relationship, family problems will become more important. A lot more emphasis has been laid on these now. Nearly 75% of my predictions have come true. As a physician, I am not trying to claim Nostradamus status.

*   *   *

I was planning to meet the miracle man originally from Hull and now living in Hampshire, Bob Weighton, who got into the Guinness Book as the world's oldest living man on 29 March 2020 at the age of 112. Bob also trotted the world. He had been a teacher most of his working life starting in Taiwan and Canada before settling back in the UK in 1939. I had met 122 year-old Jeanne Calment and 111 year-old Henry Allingham. Because of social distancing and travel regulations due to Corona virus, I could not meet Bob in person. He commented, "I'm very pleased I've been able to live so long and make so many friends." Well done, Bob for hitting a century and remaining not out.

26

The Invisible turns Invincible

Venienti Occurite Morbo

[Meet the disease as it approaches]

Persius, Roman Poet (AD 34-62)

Nostradamus, the 16th century French physician and astrologer wrote the book *Les Prophéties,* a prediction of future events. He predicted the plague of the 21st century, which turned out to be the Coronavirus.

In April 2009, H1N1 strain, the Swine Flu started in Mexico and in three months became a pandemic killing 18,200 people. Dr Bruce Aylward, head of the joint WHO-Chinese mission on the coronavirus outbreak, warned back in January, 'This is a rapidly escalating epidemic in different places that we have got to tackle super-fast to prevent a pandemic'.

All on a sudden, the word 'Coronavirus' is at the forefront of everybody's minds, thoughts and lips all around the world. In the year 2020, it has affected the entire globe except Antarctica. The dam has burst threatening the global community. This is the *Battle of Armageddon* - **Microbe** versus **Mankind**, the Third World War. The WHO has declared it as a pandemic affecting the whole world.

First of all, the Chinese Nation needs to be congratulated. As soon as the outbreak occurred, they took pro-active, drastic and draconian steps - put the city in quarantine, outlawed public gatherings, issued face masks for everybody, built a 5000-bed hospital at breath-taking speed in 10 days. Following these, they banned the sale of wild animals and sanitised bank notes. Most recently, Minivision Tech, a company in Nanjing, has developed software integrating infrared temperature scan, facial recognition and mask recognition. China has been doing minimal talking and maximum actions. The result is that new cases are steadily falling in China. That is clear evidence of an aggressive public health policy.

Here in the UK, in early stages, we have been doing lot of talking. Now, the country is in lockdown with essential activities being carried out affecting everybody with tremendous social and economic impacts beyond imagination. Until now, the death toll in the UK is about 10,000. Sir Jeremy Farrar, director of the Wellcome Trust, said, "The UK is likely to be certainly one of the worst - if not the worst affected country in Europe."

To start with, the advice from different sources have been variable and contradictory, leaving the health professionals and public in a state of confusion. As the labour peer Lord Campbell-Savours put it the advice is **'totally and utterly inadequate'**. If the outbreak were to commence here first, we would still be debating the issues taking into consideration patient choice, personal freedom, human rights and so on until the funeral directors reach a stage when they show the white flag of meltdown.

The main thrust of the advice has been hand washing for 20 seconds. A full-time GP sees 200 patients per week. He has to be washing his hands for nearly two hours. What about the patients? They keep their hands on the consultation table. The virus can stay on surfaces alive for many hours or days depending on the nature of the surface. What about the public? Shops, offices, banks, buses and trains – how can all these people keep washing their hands? The most common symptoms are flu-like cough and cold, which spreads easily by droplet infection. On an average, 3-5% of the public have a cough or cold at any given time. Where do we draw the line?

In 1665, during the Great Plague, many doctors fled London while the apothecaries stuck to their tasks. According to Pepys ' ... *this disease is making us more cruel to one another than if we were dogs'*.

The sight of the Prime Minister, the democratically elected leader in intensive care treatment, was a heart-stopping moment in the nation's diary. This clearly showed that the virus has no boundaries and we all are in danger. The craze for exotic holidays, expensive cars, Rolex watches, diamond jewellery etc have gone out through the window. We now exist in a mystifying cloud of uncertainty, perplexity and fear gripping the nation and the world, making us think deeply how suddenly within a blink of the eyes, the boundary wall between life and death collapses in our midst.

The saying 'we are all in this together' also means that we all are suffering directly and indirectly together. There has been a sense of unification among all, irrespective of age, sex, race, religion and politics. Let us draw some positives from this pandemic to put our domestic petty squabbles aside and work together for the common good, since the world has shrunk very small and life is too short.

We must be willing to let go of the life we have planned, so as to have the life that is waiting for us.'

EM Foster

Epilogue

The best sports I like are cricket and tennis. I noticed that although players start as brilliant sportsmen around 17 or 18 and do wonderfully well for a few years, by around 30, most of them are not fit for the purpose or retired. But being a doctor, you can go on as long as your health permits you to do the job. It is like vintage wine, the older and mature, one gets better. Medicine is a trade tempered with professionalism. With traditional values on one side and commercialism on the other, modern GPs serve both Aesculapius and Mammon. A medical epigram says, 'One-quarter of *saviour* and three-quarters of *saviour-faire*, makes the successful practitioner'. Looking back, if I had the chance to rehearse and play my roles in life, I might have done better.

Throughout my career, I have been fighting for my professional brethren, especially who were in distress, however strange and remote they are, in defence of fairness and justice. I have tackled things with trenchant wit and damning forthrightness. My service spanning over four decades, has been to the medical profession, local community, society and to humanity. Socrates (469-399 B C) said, 'I am a citizen, not of Athens or Greece, but of the world'. I have always felt as a citizen of Planet Earth.

This is Easter time. The Pope has just delivered the *Urbi et Orbi* (to the City and the World) message. As a humble mortal, I am delivering my story to the City (Hull) and the World.

Acknowledgements

My hearty gratitude to:

Mary (wife)

Thomas (son)

Rowena (daughter)

James (son-in-law)

Theresa (mother)

Dr Guy Clayton, GP

Dr John Zachariah, ex-GP

All my patients

The community of Hull

Editors & Proprietors of – *GP*, *PULSE*, *DOCTOR*, *BMA News review*, *Yorkshire Medicine*, *Scottish Medicine*

Printed in Poland
by Amazon Fulfillment
Poland Sp. z o.o., Wrocław